Learning from Bristol:

The Department of Health's Response to the
Report of the Public Inquiry into children's heart
surgery at the Bristol Royal Infirmary
1984-1995

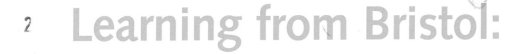

Presented to Parliament by the Secretary of State for Health
by Command of Her Majesty
January 2002

LONDON: TSO
£22.75

Cm 5363

In June 1998, the then Secretary of State for Health, the Right Honourable Frank Dobson MP, announced the establishment of an inquiry into the management of the care of children receiving complex cardiac surgery at the Bristol Royal Infirmary (BRI) between 1984 and 1995. The Inquiry was asked not only to reach conclusions about the events at Bristol, but also to make recommendations, drawn from its analysis of those events, which could help secure high quality care across the NHS. The Report of the Inquiry was published on 18 July 2001.

First and foremost, I would like to thank Professor Sir Ian Kennedy, Chairman of the Inquiry and his Panel for their meticulous account of what happened at the BRI and for the far reaching recommendations they have drawn for the NHS as a whole. The Report provides a powerful analysis of the flaws and failures of the organisation and culture, not only at the BRI in the years in question, but of the wider NHS at that time. The NHS of the 1980s and 1990s failed to keep pace with changes in society and, in particular, to reflect the views of patients and to build a service designed around their needs.

In framing the recommendations Professor Kennedy and his Panel acknowledge the progress that has been made in recent years. The vision and initiatives set out in *The NHS Plan*, launched in July 2000, and the additional resources which have been made available, set us clearly on the road that Professor Kennedy describes. But he also gives us a Report with a bigger ambition: to build a new culture, of trust not blame, within the NHS - a health service where there is greater partnership between patients and professionals; where lines of accountability are clear and where there is openness about mistakes; where services are designed from the patient's point of view and where safety for patients always comes first.

We do not underestimate the scale of this ambition. Meeting it is a challenge the Government accepts. It is a challenge we have already accepted in our own ambition to create a modern health service.

i

The Department of Health's Response to the Report of the Public Inquiry into children's heart surgery at the Bristol Royal Infirmary 1984-1995

It will take time and commitment from all who work with and for the NHS. We accept most of the recommendations and work is already underway to implement them. Others will shape the direction of our thinking in key areas. In a few cases we propose taking a different route to achieve a similar end. This document sets out our approach.

Alan Milburn
Secretary of State for Health

1. The BRI Inquiry Report provides us with a powerful analysis of the organisation and culture of the NHS in the years up to 1995. It highlights poor organisation, failure of communication, lack of leadership, paternalism and a 'club culture' and a failure to put patients at the centre of care. It draws attention to the lack of standards for evaluating performance in the NHS and for assessing the quality of care, and a lack of clarity about where the responsibility for such assessment lay, at both the local and national level. The failure to accord children's services a sufficient priority in Bristol and elsewhere in the NHS resulted in the unnecessary death and damage of a number of very young children. They were failed by the system that was supposed to make them well.

2. We accept that analysis. Without reservation we accept the broad principles upon which the Kennedy Report is based. We are seeking to develop an NHS where there is a culture of openness and honesty; where all who work in and for the NHS share the common purpose of delivering high quality, safe health care; and where patients and staff work in genuine partnership.

3. Our vision for the NHS was set out in *The NHS Plan*. We are pleased to see that the Kennedy Report recognises and acknowledges the significant contribution the Plan will make towards realising the recommendations of the Inquiry Report.

4. This calls, as the Kennedy Report recognises, for a new relationship between government and the NHS and between the NHS and patients. We recognise that the NHS needs fundamental reform if we are to deliver a high quality, patient centred service for the twenty first century. Until 1997 the Department of Health was both the headquarters and the regulator of the NHS. In the past there were no national standards: different levels of care and services were provided in different parts of the country. And there was uncertainty about where clinical and managerial responsibilities began and ended. As a result there were confused accountabilities and a lottery of care for the individual patient. Patients, faced with poor services locally, had no choice other than to wait for treatment or to opt to pay for treatment instead of it being provided by the NHS.

1

The Department of Health's Response to the Report of the Public Inquiry into children's heart surgery at the Bristol Royal Infirmary 1984-1995

5. Since 1997 we have established new independent standard setting and inspecting bodies – the Commission for Health Improvement (CHI) and the National Institute for Clinical Excellence (NICE) – outside the Department of Health. There are new bodies too – the National Patient Safety Agency (NPSA) and the National Clinical Assessment Authority (NCAA) – to tackle poor clinical practice where it has been identified. Through National Service Frameworks, national standards are in place for the first time. Through the NHS Modernisation Agency there is help for NHS organisations to improve performance. And there is more information being provided than ever before about local health service performance with rewards and intervention where appropriate.

6. *The NHS Plan* sought to build on these developments to give a new direction to the health service. The Inquiry report adds further impetus still. Today, then, the role of the Department of Health is no longer to run the NHS as if it were a mid-twentieth century nationalised industry. Instead, within the context of clear national standards that ensure fairness and quality, we are moving towards an NHS where resources and responsibilities are located in front line services which are innovative and responsive to the needs of patients. Care will be provided through a number of providers – some public, some private - delivered and inspected against those clear national standards, and all providing NHS care to NHS patients according to NHS principles. Patients will not just have more information and a greater say over local services, but more choice over who provides their care.

7. This will leave the Department of Health to set the overall framework for regulation and inspection wherever NHS care is delivered to ensure these arrangements are working to the benefit of patients, to distribute resources fairly to meet health needs and to ensure proper accountability. Regulation will be undertaken by independent bodies working to a framework of standards drawn up by patients, professionals, health service and government. Information on clinical and organisational performance will be produced independent of both government and the NHS. This more clear cut division of responsibility will tackle precisely the confusion that underpinned much of the Bristol tragedy.

8. Specifically, this far reaching change to how the NHS is run requires us to apply the Prime Minister's 4 principles of public sector reforms:

    *   high national standards and clear accountability;

    *   devolution of power and resources to the front line to give those professionals who deliver services the freedom to innovate;

- increased flexibility for staff to cut across out-moded professional barriers; and

- a greater range of alternative service providers and choice for the patient.

This will entail:

- devolution of management responsibility to front line staff through the creation of Primary Care Trusts (PCTs) and Strategic Health Authorities through the NHS Reform and Health Care Professions Bill;

- these NHS bodies to work within a framework of standards which will include the continuing development of National Service Frameworks through joint working between the NHS, the professions, patients and the Department together with the setting of evidence based standards for day to day clinical practice by NICE;

- a more independent role for NICE to set evidence based standards for day to day clinical practice, and make recommendations on the clinical cost effectiveness of new therapies for introduction into the NHS;

- in the short-term, a strengthened inspection role for CHI working with the Social Services Inspectorate and National Care Standards Commission as appropriate to give the public an independent assurance that each provider of NHS services has proper quality assurance and quality improvement mechanisms in place. We will take further steps at the earliest opportunity to rationalise the number of bodies inspecting and regulating health and social care;

- the NPSA to establish a single national system of reporting and analysis of adverse events and near misses which occur within the NHS, and to ensure that effective learning takes place to make the NHS a safer place for patients;

- the NCAA to help NHS employers assess the small minority of 'poorly performing doctors' and make recommendations about whether and under what circumstances they will continue to practise in the NHS;

- the establishment of a new Council for the Quality of Health Care to provide greater co-ordination of these bodies;

- the establishment of a new Council for the Regulation of Health Care Professionals to strengthen and co-ordinate the system of professional self-regulation; and

- the establishment through legislation of Patients' Forums in every PCT and NHS Trust, and the Commission for Patient and Public Involvement in Health to set standards and provide training and guidance to build capacity for greater community involvement in the health service.

9. The continuing improvement of services will be supported by the work of the NHS Modernisation Agency and NHS Leadership Centre in spreading good practice and developing leadership. All the bodies involved will have a responsibility to ensure the quality of services and the safety of the public. They will work with the clinical professions to ensure that doctors, nurses and other staff are supported to provide high quality care and are held to account for their performance. In addition, in the spirit of partnership on which the NHS in the future will be based, the representatives of patients and the professions will be involved at all levels in advising on strategy, inspection and regulation, and the delivery of services.

10. In taking this approach, the Government is not only endorsing the Kennedy Report's arguments for a separation of the Department of Health's roles in management and regulation but is taking these arguments a stage further.

Developing a high quality modern health service

11. In responding to the challenge set by the Kennedy Report the key tasks which lie ahead of us are to:

- put patients at the centre of the NHS;

- improve children's health care services;

- set, inspect and monitor the standards of care (the roles of CHI, NICE and NPSA);

- ensure the safety of care;

- develop a health service which is well led and managed;

- improve the regulation, education and training of health care professionals;

- improve the quality, reliability and range of information which supports decision making and strengthen the monitoring of performance; and

- involve patients and the public in health care.

Putting patients at the centre of the NHS

12. We are committed to changing attitudes in the way care is delivered. We want to develop a culture of openness, honesty and trust; to ensure that patients have the information they need to make informed choices; and to enable patients to become equal partners with health care professionals in making decisions about treatment and care.

13. Our programme of reform will include:

- more information provided to patients on how local health services compare with others and greater choice for patients over where they are treated;

- a consent process which engages patients fully in decisions about their care;

- an Expert Patient Programme to support the development of partnerships between clinicians and patients from late 2001;

- from April 2003, a National Knowledge Service for the NHS to support the delivery of high quality information for patients and staff;

- the establishment of Patient Advice and Liaison Services (PALS) within every Trust from April 2002 to assist patients in managing and accessing information;

- by the summer of 2002, guidelines about sharing information with patients and parents of young children;

- a review of bereavement services;

- publication of a Code of Practice on communicating with families about post-mortems in January 2002; and

- a reformed NHS complaints procedure by December 2002.

Improving children's health care services

14.   We agree with Professor Kennedy that there should be stronger leadership and integration at all levels in dealing with issues relating to children. Over the last 4 years we have begun to take steps to ensure that high quality and safe services are designed to meet the particular needs of children. These include several cross-government initiatives such as Sure Start and the appointment of a National Clinical Director for Children.

15.   Our programme of action, includes:

- a continued high level focus on children's issues across government;

- a senior member of staff with responsibility for children's services in every Strategic Health Authority, PCT and NHS Trust;

- children's health services designed to meet the particular needs of the children who use them and their families. The National Service Framework module on hospital care for children will be published during 2002;

- greater integration of primary, community, acute and specialist health care across professional and agency boundaries - including closer working with social services;

- clear standards against which providers of services are inspected as part of the Children's National Service Framework;

- paediatric training in an appropriate centre for all staff operating on children;

- parents fully engaged in decisions about their child's treatment and care; and

- a review by the Paediatric and Congenital Cardiac Services Review of specialist cardiac services for children. It will report in 2002.

Setting, inspecting and monitoring the standards of care – the roles of CHI, NICE and NPSA

16. We agree with Professor Kennedy that the framework for setting, delivering and monitoring standards should be made more explicit. We also agree that those bodies which assure the quality of care in the NHS should be at arm's length from the Department. However, we also believe that for standards to be achievable the bodies which assure quality must operate within a broadly agreed framework of priorities set by government, working with patients, professionals and the NHS against the overall level of resourcing available for the NHS.

17. Our future programme of action, through legislation where necessary, will include:

    * setting of clear standards through NICE and the National Service Frameworks;

    * NHS bodies being directed to fund treatments recommended by NICE from January 2002;

    * NICE guidance will no longer need the approval of the Secretary of State for Health before dissemination;

    * reinforcement of the independence of CHI in the NHS Reform and Health Care Professions Bill;

    * strengthening of CHI to take on the role of inspection of NHS organisations and service providers against the standards set for the NHS;

    * swift action where CHI identifies significant problems or where patient safety is compromised, including the imposition of 'special measures';

    * the establishment of the Office for Information on Health Care Performance as part of CHI to monitor clinical performance and to publish regular performance indicators on all NHS Trusts and PCTs; and

    * the production of an annual report by CHI on the quality of NHS services which the Secretary of State will lay before Parliament.

7

The Department of Health's Response to the Report of the Public Inquiry into children's heart surgery at the Bristol Royal Infirmary 1984-1995

Ensuring the safety of care

18.   Patient safety is at the heart of our agenda for improving the quality of NHS services. In line with the findings of *An Organisation with a Memory* and the blueprint outlined in *Building a Safer NHS for Patients* we have established the NPSA to develop a national system for reporting and analysing adverse events and 'near misses'. In addition, we are fully committed to minimising the number of adverse events occurring, for example, when a clinician undertakes a procedure for the first time or when new interventional procedures are introduced.

19.   We recognise that the current system for dealing with clinical negligence claims is slow and will therefore publish a White Paper early in 2002 setting out our plans for reform.

20.   Our programme of action also includes:

- the establishment of a single national system of reporting adverse events and 'near misses' through the NPSA during 2002;

- analysis of the data collected by the NPSA which will feed back lessons quickly to the NHS and elsewhere;

- guidance on root cause analysis to help Trusts analyse adverse events;

- work with the Design Council to identify opportunities for design solutions to safety problems;

- strengthened accountability arrangements and supervision responsibilities through job plans for consultants to ensure that junior doctors are properly supported and supervised when undertaking new procedures;

- transfer of responsibility to NICE for providing the oversight and scrutiny needed for the introduction of new interventional procedures;

- guidance for NHS Trusts on the local systems they will need for managing new interventional techniques; and

- through the consent to treatment initiative, ensuring that patients are told when their treatment is of an experimental nature.

21.   We need to ensure not only that the NHS workforce is well resourced in terms of numbers but also that there are training and development opportunities for staff to equip them with the necessary skills for a modern NHS. We are taking steps to increase the number of doctors, nurses and therapists. Through the work of the NHS Modernisation Agency's Leadership Centre and the NHS University (NHSU), we will equip board members, managers and health professionals with the skills needed to ensure effective governance and strong leadership.

22.   Our programme of action will include:

- increases in the number of staff – by 2004 there will be
  - 7,500 more consultants;
  - 2,000 more GPs;
  - 20,000 more nurses; and
  - 6,500 more therapists;

- the establishment of the NHSU from 2003;

- the support and development of leaders throughout the NHS by the NHS Modernisation Agency's Leadership Centre and the NHSU;

- all non-executive and chair appointments to Trust boards made by the NHS Appointments Commission;

- an executive director development programme from January 2002;

- clinical director and medical director development programmes from January 2002;

- an induction guide for non-executive directors to be introduced in 2002;

- mentors available for NHS Trust and PCT chairmen;

- contract changes which make more explicit the expectations placed on NHS staff by their employing NHS Trusts and PCTs; and

- through consultant appraisal, revalidation and re-registration, regular reassessment of professionals' competence both clinically and for any management duties.

Strengthening the regulation and developing the education and training of health care professionals

23. We agree with Professor Kennedy that a single body should regulate each health care profession and that there should be an overarching Council to co-ordinate those bodies, accountable to Parliament. We also agree that more needs to be done to ensure the quality of NHS management.

24. We are committed to widening access to medical schools and supporting people from non-traditional backgrounds to move into medicine. We also agree that there should be more opportunities for different health care professions to share learning and that more emphasis should be placed upon the non-clinical aspects of care, such as communication skills, in the education, training and development of those working within the NHS.

25. We envisage that appraisal will become an essential component of reflective practice and the systems which help to assure competence, quality and the safety of care. We are already committed to revalidation and are working with the General Medical Council (GMC) to introduce revalidation for all doctors.

26. Our future programme of action will include:

    - a new Council for the Regulation of Health Care Professionals to strengthen and co-ordinate the system of professional self-regulation;

    - reform of the current arrangements for the regulation of individual health care professions so that patients will be at the heart of professional regulation;

    - consultation on a new core contract for NHS senior managers, and a mandatory code of conduct;

    - wider access to medical schools by 2002 and an increase in the number of places by 2005;

    - greater public involvement in the selection of those entering training as health care professionals;

    - a new core curriculum to be introduced during 2002;

- common learning programmes across all Higher Education Institutions by 2004;

- giving priority to non-clinical aspects of care in the education, training and continuing development of those working in the NHS;

- the establishment of the Medical Education Standards Board to set standards for post-graduate medical education and training;

- investment in Continuing Professional Development;

- appraisal for all doctors;

- support for the GMC's revalidation for all doctors. We will encourage its extension to all health care professionals;

- the introduction of new criteria for NHS Clinical Excellence Awards in 2002 which will provide greater incentives for high quality, patient centred practice;

- new guidance on disciplinary procedures to support local employers in dealing with breaches of the relevant professional code by a health care professional; and

- support for the NCAA to assist NHS Trusts and PCTs when concerns about a doctor's practice first arise and before patients are harmed.

Improving information for decision making and strengthening the monitoring of performance

27. We recognise that at the moment patients and clinicians do not always get the information they need. We are committed to the development of effective systems of monitoring clinical care through local audit and through national surveillance.

28. The introduction of electronic patient records by 2005 will act as the building block for the other information the NHS needs in order to monitor quality. In the meantime we are improving and making better use of Hospital Episode Statistics (HES) data, publishing headline performance indicators for health authorities and NHS Trusts and developing a series of high quality national clinical audits.

11

The Department of Health's Response to the Report of the Public Inquiry into children's heart surgery at the Bristol Royal Infirmary 1984-1995

29.   Our future programme of action will include:

-   published data on the clinical performance of consultants and their units/teams for use by both clinicians and patients;

-   by April 2004, publication of 30 day mortality rates for the previous two years for every cardiac surgeon in England. From April 2005 annual publication on a rolling three-year basis for each centre and for each cardiac surgeon;

-   a co-ordinated approach to collecting data through the introduction of electronic patient records by 2005;

-   better use of HES data by linking hospital data to Office for National Statistics (ONS) mortality data from April 2002;

-   "star ratings" to compare the performance of NHS organisations against national targets – through the CHI Office of Information on Health Care Performance from 2002;

-   national audits in each of the clinical priority areas of *The NHS Plan*;

-   a directory of clinical audit databases from 2002; and

-   strengthening of the clinical coding function.

Involving patients and the public in health care

30.   We agree that the voices of citizens, patients and their carers should be on the inside, influencing every level of service. This means changing not only the culture of the NHS but also the mechanisms through which patients and the public get their voices heard. The Health and Social Care Act 2001 puts in place the building blocks for greater public involvement. We will build on this.

31.   Our programme for action includes:

-   establishing, through the NHS Reform and Health Care Professions Bill, Patients' Forums in every PCT and NHS Trust. Made up of local people, Forums will protect and promote patient and carer interests in the NHS by representing their views to NHS Trusts and PCTs, sitting on Trust boards, and by scrutinising local services;

- setting up the Commission for Patient and Public Involvement in Health, to set standards and provide training and guidance and build capacity within local communities for greater community involvement;

- introducing a patient survey programme from 2001 to inform local decision making;

- requiring every NHS Trust and PCT to publish an annual Patient Prospectus to demonstrate how the public have been involved and the effect of that involvement; and

- establishing a Citizens' Council to advise NICE on the values inherent in its decisions and guidance on treatments.

Conclusions

32. Bristol was a turning point in the history of the NHS. We are determined that some good can come from the tragedy that took place there. Indeed, the success of paediatric and adult heart surgery at the BRI today is not just a testament to the magnificent efforts of staff there but also a demonstration of the ability of the NHS to improve services for patients even in the most difficult of circumstances. This response to the Bristol Inquiry seeks to build a better health service for patients everywhere.

33. The next 10 chapters describe in detail the Government's response to the BRI Inquiry report. Annex A summarises our response to each recommendation.

INTRODUCTION: OUR COMMITMENT TO A HIGH QUALITY MODERN HEALTH SERVICE

This chapter sets out the relationship between the Department of Health and the National Health Service and sets the context for delivery of a high quality modern health service.

1.1   The BRI Inquiry Report provides us with a powerful analysis of the organisation and culture of the NHS in the years up to 1995. It highlights poor organisation, failure of communication, lack of leadership, paternalism and a 'club culture' and a failure to put patients at the centre of care. It draws attention to the lack of standards for evaluating performance in the NHS and for assessing the quality of care, and a lack of clarity about where the responsibility for such assessment lay, at both the local and national level. The failure to accord children's services a sufficient priority in Bristol and elsewhere in the NHS resulted in the unnecessary death and damage of a number of very young children. They were failed by the system that was supposed to make them well.

1.2   The Report of the BRI Inquiry sets out a vision in which the patient should be at the heart of the NHS and should be entitled to:

- respect and honesty;

- care in a setting which is well led;

- competent health care professionals;

- care which is safe;

- care of an appropriate standard; and

- inclusion and involvement in the NHS, both as patients and members of the public.

1.3 In delivering such a service the Inquiry is clear that safety should be central to all that is done and that organisational structures and systems should be designed to deliver safe, high quality services in an atmosphere of honesty and openness. It emphasises that securing high quality services encompasses not only technical skills and competence and the system in which they are practised, but it must move beyond those to include the attitudes which those in the NHS bring to their work. Attitude, respect and honesty and the partnership between patients and professionals are critical factors in changing the NHS culture to one where safety and quality are paramount.

Our vision for the NHS

1.4 We accept without reservation the broad principles upon which the Kennedy Report is based. We wish to move to an NHS where there is a culture of openness and honesty; where all who work in and for the NHS share the common purpose of delivering high quality, safe health care; and where the patient and health care staff work in genuine partnership.

1.5 Our vision for the NHS was set out in some detail in *The NHS Plan,* published in July 2000, and we are pleased to see that the Kennedy Report recognises and acknowledges the significant contribution *The NHS Plan* will make towards realising the recommendations of the Inquiry Report. The Report also recognises the work that has been done over the last five years to put quality centre stage in the NHS. New policies, new systems and new safeguards for patients are being implemented - work which has been undertaken jointly by the Government, the NHS and the health professions.

1.6 We are addressing the underfunding of the NHS and the March 2000 Budget settlement means that the NHS will grow by one half in cash terms and by one third in real terms in just 5 years. In addition we have recently announced a further billion pounds for health care across the UK for 2002/3. *The NHS Plan* commits us to an unparalleled increase in the number of staff and they are the key to delivering the quality improvements we seek. But we know that investment has to be accompanied by reform and the NHS has to be redesigned around the needs of the patient. Reform will address those issues that really affect patients and we have a range of proposals to empower patients to have a greater say in their care and the development of their local services.

1.7 Reform will break down the demarcations between different professional groups and organisations. Reform will free front line staff to use their skills to redesign services and improve performance.

1.8 The analysis in the Kennedy Report demonstrates the urgent need for fundamental review and reform of the relationship between government, the medical profession and the public and the nature of the structural framework which supports that relationship. The establishment of the NHS was based on an implicit understanding that government should set the budget for the NHS and the policy framework, and doctors should take responsibility for providing services and ensuring high standards. Reflecting the spirit of the times, the role of the public was limited to paying for the NHS through taxes, while patients had a largely passive role and deferred to expert judgement.

1.9 The world has changed. The public expects public services to match the standards they experience in other areas of their lives. Patients are more questioning and challenging of professionals and better informed about health and health services. They are also less willing to accept that doctor always knows best, although public trust in the medical profession remains high. Doctors have recognised that the days of untrammelled clinical freedom are over and that regulation of standards needs to be strengthened. And government has taken a more active role in promoting quality and ensuring that services are safe and effective.

1.10 The NHS after Bristol needs to be based on a new relationship that reflects these changes. That relationship must be one of partnership in which each of the partners has responsibilities as well as rights. Patients have a right to be involved in decision making and to have access to information to support decision making. They have the right to expect that professionals will act in their best interests by actively seeking their consent to treatment and being open when things go wrong. Patients also have a responsibility to treat professionals with respect and to use services appropriately. They have a responsibility to accept that mistakes will sometimes be made and that professionals should not necessarily be blamed when errors are made, provided that they are working to the best of their ability and within their competence. And they have a responsibility to adopt appropriate lifestyles and act on the professional advice they are given.

1.11 For their part, doctors have a responsibility to treat patients with dignity and respect and to work as part of a team with other clinical and non-clinical colleagues to deliver the best possible care. They have a responsibility to keep up to date in areas relevant to the service they provide, to participate in audit and clinical governance arrangements and to reflect on their own practice in order to promote a high quality service. They have a right to be valued by government and patients for the work they do. Doctors also have a right to work within a framework that enables them to exercise their professional skills and judgement, provided that they supply information about their practice for audit purposes.

1.12 Government has a responsibility to facilitate partnership between doctors and patients, and to allocate sufficient resources to enable the NHS to meet contemporary expectations. In turn, government has a right to expect doctors to develop effective systems of self-regulation and to play their part in steering and managing the NHS at all levels.

Establishing a clear framework of roles and responsibilities

Recommendation 38

The DoH's roles in relation to the NHS must in future be made explicit. The DoH should have two roles. It should be the headquarters of the NHS. It should also establish an independent framework of regulation which will assure the quality of the care provided in and funded by the NHS, and the competence of healthcare professionals.

1.13 Government has a responsibility for establishing a framework of standards and a system of regulation which clarifies for patients what they can expect and gives them effective management, leadership and professional accountability. In the past there were no national standards; there was almost complete professional autonomy for clinicians; and different levels of care and service were provided in different parts of the country. As a result there were confused accountabilities and a lottery of care for the individual patient.

1.14 What we propose, and set out in more detail through this Response, is a much clearer framework for the NHS. There will be explicit national standards, developed in partnership with the professions and patients, that apply across all parts of the country; there will be independent inspection of those standards, with clear programmes of action to remedy problems and incentives to reward and encourage progress; and there will be clear lines of accountability from front line delivery through to the Department of Health.

17

The Department of Health's Response to the Report of the Public Inquiry into children's heart surgery at the Bristol Royal Infirmary 1984-1995

1.15 The Kennedy Report proposes that the role of the Department of Health should be twofold: to act as the headquarters of the NHS; and to establish an independent framework of regulation to assure the quality of care provided in and funded by the NHS and the competence of health care professionals. This proposal has led us to undertake a fundamental re-evaluation of the roles and responsibilities of the Department of Health, NHS organisations and the bodies which have been established to regulate the quality of health care.

1.16 We believe that the Department of Health has the essential role of supporting the Secretary of State in setting the overall direction for the NHS and ensuring that there are appropriate arrangements in place for its management, standard setting, inspection, improvement and accountability. This role involves:

- setting expectations and direction. This encompasses determining strategy, policies, standards and priorities; negotiating levels of public spending, allocating resources and deciding major investments;

- ensuring the integrity of the whole system. This includes ensuring the consistency of application of new technologies and therapies across the NHS; securing integrated information systems; and making sure that developmental support is provided through the NHS Modernisation Agency and the NHS University;

- maintaining and developing the values of the NHS. The NHS represents one of the most important set of values within British society. Whilst the diverse health care institutions will be responsible for service delivery, the Department will be responsible for the development of the overall value system; and

- securing accountability for funding and performance. This includes ensuring that there are arrangements for performance assessment and inspection and maintaining a line of accountability to Parliament for public expenditure.

1.17 The Department's role in overseeing the NHS is to make sure that all these functions are undertaken and that the bodies concerned work together to provide a consistent overall framework for the NHS. It need not - and should not - do them all itself. For public services today to command public confidence they have to give greater control to the people who deliver them and greater choice to those who use them. In particular we are now bringing in changes to:

- devolve management responsibility as far as possible out of the Department to the doctors, nurses, managers and other staff working at the front line of services;

- introduce better arrangements for independent inspection, monitoring and assessment of performance;

- strengthen professional regulation;

- create greater openness with and involvement of the public; and

- provide better information for patients to strengthen choice.

Management arrangements and accountability

1.18 We propose to devolve management responsibility to front line staff through the NHS Reform and Health Care Professions Bill by:

- creating PCTs throughout the country to become the lead NHS organisations in assessing need, planning and securing all health services and improving health. They will forge new partnerships with local communities and lead the NHS contribution to joint work with local government and other partners. They will be able to focus clearly on individual patients and populations. By 2003/04 they will have responsibility for spending 75% of NHS resources.

- making PCTs and existing NHS Trusts accountable to the 28 new Strategic Health Authorities which will replace the existing 95 health authorities.

- enabling Strategic Health Authorities to step back from service planning and commissioning to lead the strategic development of the local health service and performance manage PCTs and NHS Trusts on the basis of local accountability agreements. They will agree annual delivery agreements with the Department for managing the whole health care system within their area, with specified outcomes for improvements in performance. For the first time the NHS will have a clear management and accountability structure which embraces all its parts.

Standard setting

1.19 The public are entitled to know that clear standards have been set and will apply across the whole NHS, regardless of location; that there will be effective and independent scrutiny of local delivery against these standards; and that there will be clear lines of accountability and responsibility throughout the service for the delivery of a safe, high quality service. We share this view with the Inquiry Panel.

1.20 The programme of modernisation in the NHS set in train since 1997 has for the first time introduced a comprehensive framework for quality for all NHS bodies, including mechanisms to set standards, and to assess and inspect performance. A duty has been placed on local NHS Trusts through the Health Act 1999 to assure and improve the quality of the services that they provide to patients. The key mechanism for this is clinical governance.

1.21 Since 1999 we have established a number of organisations and processes to address issues of standard setting, inspection and clinical safety:

- the National Institute for Clinical Excellence (NICE) to set evidence based standards for day to day clinical practice, and make recommendations on the clinical cost effectiveness of new therapies for use in the NHS;

- the continuing development of National Service Frameworks through joint working between the NHS, the professions, patients and the Department of Health;

- the Commission for Health Improvement (CHI) working with the Social Services Inspectorate and National Care Standards Commission, to give the public an independent assurance that each provider of NHS services has proper quality assurance and quality improvement mechanisms in place;

- the National Patient Safety Agency (NPSA) to establish a single national system of reporting and analysis of adverse events and near misses which occur within the NHS, and to ensure that effective learning takes place to make the NHS a safer place for patients; and

- the National Clinical Assessment Authority (NCAA) to help NHS employers assess the small minority of 'poorly performing doctors' and make recommendations about whether and under what circumstances they will continue to practise in the NHS. This should bring to an end long suspensions of doctors while investigations are undertaken and prevent late action to address the problem of 'rogue' doctors. It will also give doctors in difficulty more support and ensure that educational and practical solutions are found to their problems.

1.22 This framework provides a comprehensive approach to setting standards and assessing and improving quality. We now propose to further reinforce this framework by strengthening the independence of NICE, and by giving CHI an independent inspectoral role for NHS care, wherever it is delivered. All these bodies will together be responsible for standard setting, inspection, identifying risks and dangers to patients and providing specialist expertise to achieve improvement. We do recognise, however, the need for co-ordination and for this reason we plan to introduce a Council for the Quality of Health Care which will bring them together.

1.23 The continuing improvement of services will be supported by the work of the NHS Modernisation Agency and NHS Leadership Centre in spreading good practice and developing leadership. All the bodies involved will have a responsibility to ensure the quality of services and the safety of the public. They will work with the clinical professions to ensure that doctors, nurses and other staff are supported to provide high quality care and are held to account for their performance.

1.24 The Kennedy Report calls for the setting of standards of clinical care to be independent of the Department of Health and government and for a system of validation for health care organisations which would result in those organisations which failed to meet the required standards having their validation withdrawn. The Secretary of State is accountable to Parliament for the delivery of health services. We therefore consider that it is neither feasible nor desirable to separate the Department of Health's final responsibility for establishing the standards required of the health service from its responsibility for securing resources and from its responsibility for securing the delivery of acceptable health service in all areas of the country for all patients. We set out in Chapter 4 our approach to increasing the independence of NICE and CHI and our proposals for strengthening the system of independent inspection as an alternative to the introduction of validation.

21

The Department of Health's Response to the Report of the Public Inquiry into children's heart surgery at the Bristol Royal Infirmary 1984-1995

Professional regulation

1.25 The public has a right to know that any health care professional providing care is skilled and competent to do so. We have already signalled our intent to modernise the regulation of health care professionals in *The NHS Plan.* Our proposals are designed to replace the current fragmented arrangements with a modern framework that puts the patient at the heart of the process, and gives the public greater safeguards. Through the NHS Reform and Health Care Professions Bill we propose to establish a Council for the Regulation of Health Care Professionals to strengthen and co-ordinate the system of professional self-regulation.

Putting the patient at the centre of care

1.26 The central message of the Kennedy Report and the main theme of all our reforms is the need to put the patient at the centre of the health service and the way in which care is delivered. This applies equally to an individual's involvement in decisions about their own care and broader public involvement in planning the delivery of health care services. Patients must be offered true choices about the care they receive and where they receive it. To be able to exercise choice, patients need good information - on proposed treatments and on comparative clinical and organisational performance.

1.27 Our commitment to introducing modern IT systems, and providing easy access to validated sources of information will support this. By helping patients make choices we will ensure that PCTs and hospitals respond more directly to the needs and wishes of patients. Already over 4 million patients are being given a choice over the **time** of their treatment through the booked admissions programme. Later in 2002 we will begin introducing choice for patients over the **location** of their treatment when people who have waited for heart surgery for six months will be able to choose an alternative provider. By 2005 every patient needing hospital treatment will be helped by their GP to choose both the date and the location of that treatment. We intend to make these choices available to all NHS patients. Our aim is to create a more decentralised, more diverse, more responsive health service, capable of offering patients better services and greater choice.

1.28 Choice is also about giving the wider public more influence over how the NHS services are delivered. We are introducing a range of initiatives and mechanisms which will encourage and support patients to inform and influence the development of services. Patients will serve as members of NHS Trust boards for the first time and will be central to local decision making. Chapter 9 sets out our proposal in more detail.

1.29 Empowering patients and supporting public involvement is crucial to redress the old fashioned and unbalanced relationship between patients and services and to providing the impetus for reform in the way health care is delivered. In the twentieth century NHS patients were assumed to be passive recipients of care. In the twenty first century NHS patients will be active partners in care. In the twentieth century health service patients had little information and no choice about services. In the twenty first century health service patients will have information to make informed choices about their care. In the twentieth century health services effectively chose their patients. In the twenty first century health service patients will choose their services. This changed relationship between services and patients will put patients in the driving seat. It will make for an NHS designed around the needs and convenience of the patient. It will address precisely the structural problem of disempowered patients that underpinned the tragedies of Bristol. This crucial element of patient involvement completes the framework for the delivery of health care in which there is clarity of standards; independent assessment of performance against those standards; effective action to address identified deficiencies in performance; and a patient centred approach to the provision of a high quality, safe health care service.

1.30 There will be then a new relationship between patients and services, and between the NHS and government. Details of how we propose to implement this framework are embedded in the chapters to follow. They set out the means by which we will seek to deliver the vision and ambition given to us by the BRI Inquiry Report.

1.31 We do not always accept the means proposed by Professor Kennedy and his Panel. Sometimes we have already committed to one course of action; in other areas we propose a different solution or alternative way forward. What we do share however, are the values and the vision of an NHS where patients are at the centre of all we do, where safety is paramount and where there is a new patient centred culture in the NHS.

RESPECT AND HONESTY: PATIENTS AT THE CENTRE OF THE NHS

The Kennedy Report and this Response deal in some detail with the structures and organisations of the NHS, with the mechanism for ensuring the safety of care and the competence of the staff who work in the service. All these elements are necessary if we are to provide the high quality health service demanded by a modern society. But we must not lose sight of the individual patient at the centre of all this activity. This chapter deals with some of the issues which most clearly impact on individual choice and decision making, on the nature of the individual relationship between the patient and the professionals providing care, and on the special circumstances surrounding the family where the patient is a child.

Patient Choice

2.1 Our aim is to create a more decentralised, more diverse, more responsive health service which is capable of offering patients better services and greater choice. By helping patients make choices we will ensure that PCTs and hospitals respond more directly to the needs and wishes of patients. Over 4 million patients have already been given a choice over the **time** of their treatment through the booked admissions programme, and later this year we will begin introducing choice for patients over the **location** of their treatment when people who have waited for heart surgery for six months will be able to choose an alternative provider.

2.2 By 2005 every patient needing hospital treatment will be helped by their GP to choose both the date and the location of that treatment. Patients and doctors will be able to consider a range of options. This might include local NHS hospitals, NHS hospitals or diagnostic and treatment centres elsewhere, private hospitals, private diagnostic and treatment centres, or even hospitals overseas. They will be able to compare different waiting times at different hospitals and across different specialties. GPs and referring consultants will be able to book appointments online. By increasing patient choice in this way we are seeking to redress the old imbalance of power between patients and services and provide the impetus to reform the way health care is delivered. The nature of the relationship between the patient and health care professional is also critical. This chapter looks at the way we are supporting patients to become equal partners in making decisions about their care and treatment.

Consent

Recommendations 1, 5, 11, 13, 15, 23-26

Recommendation 1

In a patient-centred healthcare service patients must be involved, wherever possible, in decisions about their treatment and care.

Recommendation 5

Information should be tailored to the needs, circumstances and wishes of the individual.

Recommendation 11

Patients should always be given the opportunity and time to ask questions about what they are told, to seek clarification and to ask for more information. It must be the responsibility of employers in the NHS to ensure that the working arrangements of healthcare professionals allow for this, not least that they have the necessary time.

Recommendation 13

Before embarking on any procedure, patients should be given an explanation of what is going to happen and, after the procedure, should have the opportunity to review what has happened.

Recommendation 15

Patients should be told that they may have another person of their choosing present when receiving information about a diagnosis or a procedure.

Recommendation 23

We note and endorse the recent statement on consent produced by the DoH: *Reference guide to consent for examination or treatment,* 2001. It should inform the practice of all healthcare professionals in the NHS and be introduced into practice in all trusts.

Recommendation 24

The process of informing the patient, and obtaining consent to a course of treatment, should be regarded as a process and not a one-off event consisting of obtaining a patient's signature on a form.

Recommendation 25

The process of consent should apply not only to surgical procedures but also to all clinical procedures and examinations which involve any form of touching. This must not mean more forms: it means more communication.

Recommendation 26

As part of the process of obtaining consent, except when they have indicated otherwise, patients should be given sufficient information about what is to take place, the risks, uncertainties, and possible negative consequences of the proposed treatment, about any alternatives and about the likely outcome, to enable them to make a choice about how to proceed.

2.3   The Kennedy Report is clear that partnership between the patient and health care professional and the exchange and provision of information is the way forward to developing a culture of openness and honesty. We endorse that view. Elsewhere in this Response we outline our proposals for improving the quality and availability of information on clinical outcomes, which will enable patients to become equal partners in the process of decision making about their care. The Kennedy Report recognises the critical importance of giving patients the right information in ways they need and can understand. Giving consent is a process which takes time: it is not a one-off activity. It is one of the ways in which information can be used to help patients to make informed choices about their illness and its treatment. The Report recognises that we have already made progress in establishing good practice in consent as promised in *The NHS Plan*.

2.4   In March 2001 we published a *Reference Guide to Consent for Examination or Treatment* which provides clear guidance to the NHS on the legal requirements relating to consent. In July 2001 we published leaflets for patients, *Consent – what you have a right to expect,* setting out their right to be involved in their own health care decisions, and to receive the information and support they need to do so. In November 2001, we published a new model consent form and model consent policy that will give further impetus to these aims. Patients and professional groups have been involved in designing and testing out these forms.

2.5   The *Reference Guide to Consent for Examination or Treatment* has been widely distributed to health professionals. The model consent policy draws attention to the requirements of the *Reference Guide* and requires NHS organisations to consider procedural factors such as:

- when consent is sought;

- the availability of written information for patients ; and

- the availability of training for health professionals.

These will be central in determining how patients actually experience the consent process.

2.6   Both the *Reference Guide* and the model consent policy make very clear that consent should be regarded as a process, of which the signing of a consent form (where appropriate) is only the endpoint. They also make very clear that a patient's consent should always be sought before any kind of personal care or treatment is offered and there should be the opportunity for the health professional to review, with the patient, what has happened afterwards. Signing a consent form is only one way of indicating consent, and in many cases it will be perfectly acceptable for patients to indicate their consent orally or even non-verbally. In whatever form patients signal their consent, they must receive enough information in a suitable form to be able to take an informed decision, and good communication between health professionals and patients is essential in achieving this.

2.7   The new model consent forms make clear that patients should be informed of the intended benefits of the proposed procedure, any serious or frequently occurring risks, what the treatment will involve and what, if any, alternative treatments are available. Patients are encouraged to ask questions and raise any concerns that they wish both through general leaflets about consent and in the patients' notes on signing a consent form, which comprise part of the new model forms. It also encourages patients to take someone with them to the consultation if they wish, and to take the time to think about their decision and discuss it with their families if they wish. Guidance to health professionals, both in the *Reference Guide* and on the new consent forms, makes clear that any questions should be answered honestly. Both the new model consent forms and the model consent policy highlight the importance of written information being provided to back up information given face to face.

Partnership

> **Recommendations 2, 3, 16**
>
> **Recommendation 2**
> **The education and training of all healthcare professionals should be imbued with the idea of partnership between the healthcare professional and the patient.**
>
> **Recommendation 3**
> **The notion of partnership between the healthcare professional and the patient, whereby the patient and the professional meet as equals with different expertise, must be adopted by healthcare professionals in all parts of the NHS, including healthcare professionals in hospitals.**
>
> **Recommendation 16**
> **Patients should be given the sense of freedom to indicate when they do not want any (or more) information: this requires skill and understanding from healthcare professionals.**

2.8   We wholeheartedly agree with the Kennedy Report that patients should be put at the centre of care and should be the focus of team working and inter-personal care. Translating this into reality is more difficult and will take time. We are actively seeking to instil this approach in the way we educate and train professionals and other staff and in the way we teach them to communicate with patients and their families. When the Chief Medical Officer wrote to the General Medical Council in response to consultation on its revision of *Tomorrow's Doctors* he said that doctors of the future would:

- be able to engage effectively in activities to assess the quality of their services and to plan quality assurance and improvement measures;

- understand how to work in a team;

- have the communication skills necessary to underpin a true doctor and patient partnership; and

- be able to access and use data, information and evidence to assess a service or clinical intervention or to inform a clinical decision.

2.9   *Tomorrow's Doctors* is the policy document which will shape the design of undergraduate medical curricula in the years ahead. Communicating well means listening as well as telling and responding to the needs of patients in terms of the information they actually want. We have described the importance we place on developing communication skills throughout the working life of health care staff in Chapter 7.

2.10   Patients with long-term chronic conditions often have a great deal of knowledge about how to maintain or improve their health and quality of life. They can become 'experts' in their own right and have the potential to be confident partners with the medical professions in their own care. To recognise this potential and support the development of genuine partnership between clinicians and patients the Department of Health has launched the Expert Patients Programme which, from late 2001, provides user–led self management schemes for people with chronic long-term conditions.

Keeping patients informed about treatment and care

Recommendations 4 - 10, 12

Recommendation 4

Information about treatment and care should be given in a variety of forms, be given in stages and be reinforced over time.

Recommendation 5

Information should be tailored to the needs, circumstances and wishes of the individual.

Recommendation 6

Information should be based on the current available evidence and include a summary of the evidence and data, in a form which is comprehensible to patients.

Recommendation 7

Various modes of conveying information, whether leaflets, tapes, videos or CDs, should be regularly updated, and developed and piloted with the help of patients.

Recommendation 8

The NHS Modernisation Agency should make the improvement of the quality of information for patients a priority. In relation to the content and the dissemination of information for patients, the Agency should identify and promote good practice throughout the NHS. It should establish a system for accrediting materials intended to inform patients.

> **Recommendation 9**
>
> **The public should receive guidance on those sources of information about health and healthcare on the Internet which are reliable and of good quality: a kitemarking system should be developed.**
>
> **Recommendation 10**
>
> **Tape-recording facilities should be provided by the NHS to enable patients, should they so wish, to make a tape recording of a discussion with a healthcare professional when a diagnosis, course of treatment, or prognosis is being discussed.**
>
> **Recommendation 12**
>
> **Patients must be given such information as enables them to participate in their care.**

2.11 The Kennedy Report calls for good quality information for patients, relatives, carers or friends to be widely available, and in a variety of formats and media. We are creating a new National Knowledge Service for the NHS, which will provide a framework for identifying and meeting the needs for knowledge to support patient care. It will meet the needs of professionals, patients and the public for up to date, cross-referenced evidence based information by fully integrating the development of NHS knowledge systems (e.g. NHS Direct, NHS UK, the National Electronic Library for Health, Department of Health websites, emerging access technologies etc.). This is a complex development which will take time and resources, but we envisage that the National Knowledge Service will be able to offer:

- quality assured (kitemarked) patient information on a variety of diseases, conditions and treatments in different languages and aimed at a variety of educational levels;

- greater equity of access to information for everyone involved in the health care process (e.g. unlimited access to the Cochrane Library, British Medical Journal, clinical evidence); and

- wider access to information through a range of NHS public access technologies, for example, NHS Direct Information Points.

2.12 The establishment of Patient Advice and Liaison Services (PALS) within NHS Trusts and PCTs will also assist patients in managing information and in accessing information sources. The Kennedy Report acknowledges the role the NHS Modernisation Agency must play in ensuring the information which patients receive is considered in all its programmes and it will continue to monitor the patient experience together with implementing and sharing good practice. We do not accept the recommendation that patients should be provided with tape recording facilities if they wish to record a discussion with a health care professional. We believe that such a move might undermine the trust relationship between professional and patient.

2.13 In addition, to ensure that patients have access to information whilst receiving care, we have instigated the Patient Power initiative, so that bedside TV and telephones will be available in every major hospital by December 2003. As these systems become operational there is scope for providing a range of additional services to patients, for example patients (and hospital staff) may be able to access the following at the bedside terminal:

- electronic patient records;

- an information channel dedicated to providing patient information about the hospital they are in; and

- information to assist the hospital to alert the patient to safety, security and fire alarm information.

2.14 But patients also need specific information about the performance of the NHS Trust offering care and the outcomes achieved by the consultant leading their care. Chapter 8 sets out our plan for improving the range and quality of information available to patients, clinicians and managers.

Support for patients

> **Recommendations 14, 17, 18, 20**
>
> **Recommendation 14**
> Patients should be supported in dealing with the additional anxiety sometimes created by greater knowledge.
>
> **Recommendation 17**
> Patients should receive a copy of any letter written about their care or treatment by one healthcare professional to another.
>
> **Recommendation 18**
> Parents of those too young to take decisions for themselves should receive a copy of any letter written by one healthcare professional to another about their child's treatment or care.
>
> **Recommendation 20**
> The provision of counselling and support should be regarded as an integral part of a patient's care. All hospital trusts should have a well-developed system and a well-trained group of professionals whose task it is to provide this type of support and to make links to the various other forms of support (such as that provided by voluntary or social services) which patients may need.

2.15 We recognise that whilst it is right that patients and families should have access to high quality information about their illness and the procedures they face, this knowledge can in itself cause significant anxiety - a fact reflected in the Kennedy Report. We have set up a Working Group to look at how best we can make information available to patients or parents of young children. It will produce guidelines by the summer of 2002 which will also include suggestions about how patients and parents should be supported in dealing with the additional anxiety that access to greater knowledge can bring.

2.16 Health care staff are clearly central to providing this support. For example, registered nurses, midwives and health visitors all practise under a Code of Conduct which requires them to 'act at all times in such a manner as to safeguard and promote the interest of individual patients'. Their education and training prepares them to plan and deliver care for the emotional and spiritual needs of their patients as well as their physical and mental needs. These standards are reflected in the codes of practice for all other NHS professions.

2.17 PALS will also play an integral part in the provision of support. They will be introduced into every NHS Trust by April 2002 and will be accessible to patients, their families and their carers, providing advice on all aspects of NHS Trust services, including access to counselling and support. PALS pathfinders are currently set up to determine best practice guidelines. These will be issued to the NHS soon.

Bereavement services

> ### Recommendations 21, 22
>
> #### Recommendation 21
> **Every trust should have a professional bereavement service. (We also reiterate what was recommended in the Inquiry's Interim Report: 'Recommendation 13: As hospitals develop websites, a domain should be created concerned with bereavement in which all the relevant information concerning post-mortems can be set out in an appropriate manner.')**
>
> #### Recommendation 22
> **Voluntary organisations which provide care and support to patients and carers in the NHS (such as through telephone helplines, the provision of information and the organisation of self-help groups) play a very important role. Groups which meet the appropriate standards as laid down by the NHS should receive appropriate funding from the state for the contribution they make to the NHS.**

2.18 The Kennedy Report rightly highlights the need for high quality services for bereaved people. We have already accepted the Chief Medical Officer's recommendations in *The Removal, Retention and the Use of Human Organs and Tissue From Post-Mortem Examination* (January 2001) that all NHS Trusts should provide support and advice to families at the time of bereavement. Specific guidance was issued to the NHS in 1992 which recommends the scope and quality of service to be offered to bereaved people. The Department of Health has a website setting out the guidance and we are currently reviewing the quality and quantity of bereavement services throughout England.

2.19 We are developing a Code of Practice on communicating with families about post-mortems. It will include guidance on the range of information that may be required, including advice that enables families to decide whether to give consent to a hospital post-mortem, and details of the range of support that families may need at the time of bereavement. We issued the code for consultation in January 2002 as part of a broader package of measures to reinforce an approach to the retention and use of human organs and tissue after post-mortem based firmly in consent and the 'gift relationship'.

2.20   As Professor Kennedy recognises, voluntary organisations can play an important role in providing care and support to patients, carers and families. The NHS is already able to fund, or purchase under contract, care and support services from voluntary organisations as an alternative to providing such services itself and local arrangements are in place to do this.

Responding to patients when things go wrong

Recommendations 33 - 36

Recommendation 33

A duty of candour, meaning a duty to tell a patient if adverse events have occurred, must be recognised as owed by all those working in the NHS to patients.

Recommendation 34

When things go wrong, patients are entitled to receive an acknowledgement, an explanation and an apology.

Recommendation 35

There should be a clear system, in the form of a 'one-stop shop' in every trust, for addressing the concerns of a patient about the care provided by, or the conduct of, a healthcare professional.

Recommendation 36

Complaints should be dealt with swiftly and thoroughly, keeping the patient (and carer) informed. There should be a strong independent element, not part of the trust's management or board, in any body considering serious complaints which require formal investigation. An independent advocacy service should be established to assist patients (and carers).

2.21   The BRI Inquiry Report calls for patients to receive an explanation and apology when things go wrong, with complaints being dealt with swiftly and thoroughly.

2.22 We agree that staff should be open and candid about errors. Whether or not they wish to make a complaint patients are entitled to a full explanation and apology when something has gone wrong. We deal with this in more detail in Chapter 5. Under the current NHS complaints procedure every NHS Trust and PCT must have a designated complaints manager, who is readily accessible to the public.

2.23 All complaints should receive a positive and full response, with the aim of satisfying the complainants that their concerns have been heeded, and offered an apology and explanation as appropriate, referring to any remedial action that is to follow. Complainants have the right to ask for an independent review of their complaint if they remain dissatisfied with the outcome of local resolution. However, despite these procedures we recognise that there is major dissatisfaction with the current complaint processes.

2.24 We therefore issued *Reforming the NHS Complaints Procedure* in September 2001 to ask NHS staff, patient representative groups and others with an interest in the NHS complaints procedure for their views on reforming the current arrangements in order to deliver a robust high quality service that addresses the concerns of people who want to complain about NHS services. New guidance will be issued to the NHS with a view to implementing reforms to the NHS complaints procedure from late 2002. The aim will be to develop a system which:

- is responsive to the concerns of patients and their families;

- avoids defensiveness;

- provides an explanation and apology when things have gone wrong;

- is used to identify and act on systems failures and problems within the organisation;

- is used positively by NHS Trusts and PCTs as they develop into 'learning organisations'; and

- allows lessons learned to be shared nationally where appropriate.

2.25 The Health and Social Care Act 2001 already places a new duty on the Secretary of State to make arrangements for independent support to be available for people wishing to make a complaint against the NHS. Patients or carers will be able to access this service directly to assist them in making a complaint about NHS services – if this is what the patient or carer wants. We will seek to ensure that this support is provided in a way that delivers a consistent and high quality service across the country and between organisations.

Conclusion

2.26 The guiding principles of the Kennedy Report are respect for patients and honesty in the transactions between health care professionals and patients. We have already introduced a major initiative on improving the consent process; we recognise the need to provide information in a variety of forms to enable patients to develop the knowledge needed to make informed choices; and we will put in place a range of measures to help guide and support patients towards more equal relationships with those who provide their care.

2.27 Progress is being made on improving the range and quality of information available to patients, clinicians and managers through the following actions and initiatives:

- the consent process will engage patients fully in decisions about their care. The National Clinical Governance Support Team will provide training to support this;

- the Expert Patient Programme began to support the development of partnerships between clinicians and patients from late 2001. This will be available across the country from 2004;

- from April 2003 the National Knowledge Service for the NHS will, over time, support the delivery of high quality information for patients and staff;

- the establishment of PALS within every NHS Trust by April 2002 will assist patients in managing and accessing information;

- the Patient Power initiative will be available in every major hospital by December 2003;

- by the summer of 2002 guidelines will be available about sharing information with patients and parents of young children;

- a Code of Practice on communicating with families about post-mortems will be available in early 2002; and

- there will be a reformed NHS complaints procedure by the end of 2002.

The Department of Health's Response to the Report of the Public Inquiry into children's heart surgery at the Bristol Royal Infirmary 1984-1995

THE CARE OF CHILDREN

This chapter recognises the importance of providing leadership for children's services at all levels; designing and providing services to meet the health care needs of children; and the progress we have made in meeting these objectives, and in meeting the needs of children with congenital heart disease.

3.1   In considering the wider lessons of the BRI Inquiry Report for the NHS as a whole we should not lose sight of the fact that the Inquiry was established in response to significant failings and shortcomings in the way care for seriously ill children was delivered in Bristol. The Report itself laments the lack of priority given to children's services. We are committed to changing this and to ensuring that children, just like adults, are entitled to high quality, safe services designed to meet their particular needs. Children should not have to make do with services designed for adults, which are, quite simply, inappropriate for them.

3.2   We recognise and share the concerns of the Kennedy Report that children have not always had the priority within our society that they deserve and that there has not been strong enough leadership and integration for children's services. Over the last 4 years we have sought to redress this balance, although there is considerable progress still to be made. As Professor Kennedy acknowledges, we are committed to removing the inequalities in children's life chances: we are already taking steps to improve education, to reduce health inequalities and to tackle child poverty.

Responsibility for children's services

Recommendations 168 - 171

Recommendation 168

Consideration should be given to the creation of an office of Children's Commissioner in England, with the role of promoting the rights of children in all areas of public policy and seeking improvements to the ways in which the needs of children are met. Healthcare would be one of the areas covered by such a commissioner. Were such an office to be created, we would see it as being in addition to, rather than in place of, our other recommendations about the need to improve the quality of leadership in children's healthcare services.

Recommendation 169

The Cabinet Committee on Children and Young People's Services should specifically include in its remit matters to do with healthcare and health services for children and young people.

Recommendation 170

Each health authority and each primary care group or primary care trust should designate a senior member of staff who should have responsibility for commissioning children's healthcare services locally.

Recommendation 171

All trusts which provide services for children as well as adults, should have a designated executive member of the board whose responsibility it is to ensure that the interests of children are protected and that they are cared for in a paediatric environment by paediatrically trained staff.

3.3   We agree that there needs to be stronger leadership and integration at all levels in looking at issues that relate to children. To this end:

- we have appointed a Minister for Young People;

- the Cabinet Committee for Children and Young People's Services, chaired by the Chancellor of the Exchequer, is designed to give a proper focus on children at the heart of government. Every Secretary of State with responsibilities for children's issues is a member and its remit runs across the whole of government;

39

The Department of Health's Response to the Report of the Public Inquiry into children's heart surgery at the Bristol Royal Infirmary 1984-1995

- we have established a Children and Young People's Unit, reporting to the Minister for Young People, to operate across government to co-ordinate policies that will support the Prime Minister's pledge to halve child poverty in ten years. A key role for the unit is the management of the Children's Fund: £450m of additional funding over three years targeted at vulnerable children and young people as part of the Government's strategy to tackle child poverty and social exclusion;

- we have set up the Sure Start programme as part of our drive to tackle poverty and social exclusion ;

- we have created an independent Children's Rights Director (under the Care Standards Act 2000) for some of our most vulnerable children;

- a Children's Commissioner has been appointed in Wales and there is consultation underway in Northern Ireland. We will learn the lessons of these initiatives before deciding whether to appoint an English Commissioner;

- we have established a Children's Task Force to co-ordinate health and social care provision for children;

- we have announced and begun work on a National Service Framework for Children;

- we have appointed a National Clinical Director for Children to spearhead this work; and

- we have established the Paediatric and Congenital Cardiac Services Review Group to look at issues relating to the future position of this service.

3.4 This central focus needs to be reflected locally if children's interests are to be accorded sufficient priority in the planning and delivery of health services. We have therefore accepted in principle the Kennedy recommendations that each Strategic Health Authority, Primary Care Group and PCT should have a senior member of staff responsible for the planning and commissioning of local children's health care services and that each NHS Trust which provides services for children should have a designated executive director with responsibility for protecting children's interests. These recommendations will be pursued through *Shifting the Balance of Power* and the Children's National Service Framework.

Setting standards for children's health care services

Recommendation 167

A National Director for Children's Healthcare Services should be appointed to promote improvements in healthcare services provided for children.

Recommendation 172

The proposed National Service Framework (NSF) for children's healthcare services must be agreed and implemented as a matter of urgency.

Recommendation 173

The NSF should include a programme for the establishment of standards in all areas of children's acute hospital and healthcare services.

Recommendation 174

The NSF should set obligatory standards which must be observed, as well as standards to which children's services should aspire over time.

Recommendation 175

The NSF should include incentives for the improvement of children's healthcare services, with particular help being given to those trusts most in need.

Recommendation 176

The NSF must include plans for the regular publication of information about the quality and performance of children's healthcare services at national level, at the level of individual trusts, and of individual consultant units.

3.5   We have appointed Professor Al Aynsley-Green, Nuffield Professor of Child Health at the Institute of Child Health and Great Ormond Street Hospital, to the post of National Clinical Director for Children. He is leading work on the development of a National Service Framework for children. We have asked Professor Aynsley-Green to bring forward the module of work looking at standards for hospital care for children for publication this year. He has established a working group, co-chaired by Professor David Hall, President of the Royal College of Paediatrics and Child Health and Jo Williams, Director of Social Services in Cheshire, to support him in this work.

3.6 We expect the NSF to reflect some clear principles that will shape the future development of all children's services. It will give careful consideration to the Inquiry's recommendations about the configuration and organisation of children's services. It will develop care pathways to ensure greater integration between primary and secondary care. The NSF will also address the question of greater integration of services between the different sectors, including integration of health and social care services. Standards and service models will be developed around the needs of children and families. Consultation with children and young people and their families and carers will be a key part of the NSF development process. Compliance with the standards the NSF sets will not be optional. The NSF will include a strategy for implementing standards over a phased period together with an information strategy, as recommended by Professor Kennedy.

3.7 Implementation of the NSF will be consistent with our wider regime of performance management in the NHS and its system of incentives, "earned autonomy" and remedial options. We will give full consideration to targeted funding and incentive payments as recommended by Professor Kennedy where they would be the most effective way of delivering and maintaining improvement and where they are consistent with our overall approach to the NHS.

3.8 The Kennedy Report proposes a set of obligatory standards for children's services and the validation of all NHS Trusts which provide acute hospital services for children against those standards. The question of validation is considered later in this Response. The NSF will set standards which will apply to all NHS Trusts providing health services, including acute hospital services to children and will incorporate a process for ensuring those standards are met. CHI will inspect NHS Trusts against those standards and, where there are issues or concerns, it will recommend to the Secretary of State measures to address them.

Planning the future of children's health care services

Recommendation 177 - 181, 183

Recommendation 177

There must be much greater integration of primary, community, acute and specialist healthcare for children. The NSF should include strategic guidance to health authorities and trusts so that services in the future are better integrated and organised around the needs of children and their families.

Recommendation 178

Children's acute hospital services should ideally be located in a children's hospital, which should be physically as close as possible to an acute general hospital. This should be the preferred model for the future.

Recommendation 179

In the case of existing free-standing children's hospitals, particular attention must be given to ensuring that, through good management and organisation of care, children have access when needed to (a) facilities which may not routinely be found in a children's hospital and (b) specialists, the appointment of whom in a children's hospital could not be justified given the infrequent call on their services.

Recommendation 180

Consideration should be given to piloting the introduction of a system whereby children's hospitals take over the running of the children's acute and community services throughout a geographical area, building on the example of the Philadelphia Children's Hospital in the USA.

Recommendation 181

Specialist services for children should be organised so as to provide the best available staff and facilities, thus providing the best possible opportunity for good outcomes. Advice should be sought from experts on the appropriate number of patients to be treated to achieve good outcomes. In planning and organising specialist services, the requirements of quality and safety should prevail over considerations of ease of access.

Recommendation 183

After completion of a pilot exercise, all trusts which provide acute hospital services for children should be subject to a process of validation to ensure that they have appropriate child- and family-centred policies, staff, and facilities to provide a good standard of care for children. Trusts which are not so validated should not, save in emergencies, provide acute hospital services for children.

3.9   The Kennedy Report is clear that there must be greater integration of primary, community, acute and specialist health care for children and we share this view. The care of sick children needs to be seamless as they move between hospital and home and between general and highly specialist services. The NSF will reflect core *NHS Plan* values, particularly the importance of building services around the needs of service users. A key theme throughout will be the better integration of services and working in partnership, including the breakdown of unhelpful professional and agency boundaries which get in the way of delivering the best care to children.

3.10   The Kennedy Report invites us to look again at the way health care services for children are delivered and to set standards for the services offered. The NSF will consider all the available evidence on which to base its standards, including those relating to the configuration of children's hospital services, and the need for children to have access to the full range of specialist and general services. We will commission an evaluation of alternative models for the management of children's services and publish the findings as part of the NSF.

3.11   Specialist services must be organised in such a way as to deliver the best possible clinical outcomes and the Paediatric and Congenital Cardiac Services Review is already looking at these issues for cardiac care. The NSF will build on that work and will also consider tertiary services more widely, taking account of the specific recommendations of the Kennedy Report.

Financial support for patients and families

Recommendation 142

Where the interests of securing quality of care and the safety of patients require that there be only a small number of centres offering a specialist service, the requirements of quality and safety should prevail over considerations of ease of access. It is and should be the responsibility of the NHS to assist patients, and their families or carers, with the cost of transport and accommodation when they have to travel away from home to receive specialist services. Such support should not be the subject of a means test.

Recommendation 182

Where *specialist* services for children are concentrated in a small number of trusts spread throughout England, these trusts should establish Family Support Funds to help families to meet the costs arising from travelling and staying away from home. The Funds should be administered flexibly and should not be limited to those on income support or with low incomes.

3.12 As the Kennedy Report points out, organising services to deliver the highest and safest standards of care may in some cases result in families travelling away from home to be with their children. The hospital travel costs scheme ensures that no patient needing hospital treatment is denied it because they are unable to afford the cost of travel to hospital. The scheme does not include visiting costs. We recognise and share the Inquiry's view of the value of parental visits to the well-being of sick children and the value of parents being involved in their children's care, but we are also sensitive to the need for the NHS to devote as much as possible of its finite resources to funding direct patient care. We are therefore actively exploring options to support families unable to meet the additional financial burden of a child in hospital, whilst not extending it to cover all families, regardless of income. This consideration will also extend to the financial support of adults who have to travel to specialist centres for their care.

The staffing of children's health care services

Recommendations 184 - 186

Recommendation 184

Children should always (save in exceptional circumstances, such as emergencies) be cared for in a paediatric environment, and always by healthcare professionals who hold a recognised qualification in caring for children. This is especially so in relation to paediatric intensive care.

Recommendation 185

The 1991 standards for the numbers of paediatrically qualified nurses required at any given time should serve as the minimum standard and should apply where children are treated (save in emergencies). The standards should be reviewed as a matter of urgency to take account of changing patterns in the provision of acute healthcare services.

Recommendation 186

All surgeons who operate on children, including those who also operate on adults, must undergo training in the care of children and obtain a recognised professional qualification in the care of children. As a matter of priority, the GMC, the body responsible for the revalidation of doctors, should agree with the Royal College of Surgeons of England the appropriate number and range of procedures which surgeons who operate on children must undertake in order to retain their validation. This will have consequences for the way in which general surgery for children is organised.

3.13   We share Professor Kennedy's view that children should be cared for in an environment appropriate to their age, and their physical and psychological development, by health care professionals with appropriate qualifications and experience and this will be reflected in the NSF. We expect the NSF to review and update the standards issued in 1991 for the numbers of qualified paediatric nurses, but agree that in the meantime these standards should continue to apply to children in hospital.

3.14   We recognise that children's surgery requires a range of special skills and expertise and that these should be reflected in the training and qualifications of those who perform surgery on children. We agree that all surgeons who operate on children should have paediatric training or be part of a recognised training programme. This is a complex area and we will work with the Specialist Training Authority of the Medical Royal Colleges and the profession to clarify the scope of specialist paediatric surgical practice, the training requirements and the needs of non-paediatric surgeons who are required to carry out surgery on children, and the evidence based performance indicators to support the revalidation of these clinicians. We will ensure through clinical governance, appraisal and by supporting the GMC's revalidation that any doctor practising as a paediatric surgeon has all the necessary skills to do so.

Communication between health care professionals, children and their parents or carers

Recommendations 187 - 191

Recommendation 187

Parents should ordinarily be recognised as experts in the care of their children, and when their children are in need of healthcare, parents should ordinarily be fully involved in that care.

Recommendation 188

Parents of very young children have particular knowledge of their child. This knowledge must be valued and taken into account in the process of caring for the child, unless there is a good reason to do otherwise.

Recommendation 189

Children's questions about their care must be answered truthfully and clearly.

Recommendation 190

Healthcare professionals intending to care for children should be trained in the particular skills necessary to communicate with parents and with children.

Recommendation 191

Healthcare professionals should be honest and truthful with parents in discussing their child's condition, possible treatment and the possible outcome.

3.15 We agree with the Kennedy Report's view that parents are normally the experts on their own children and that they should be fully involved in their care and treatment. How to achieve a greater involvement of parents and children in planning care will be a theme of the NSF. *Consent – what you have a right to expect* emphasises the child's right to ask questions about their care and treatment and the *Reference Guide to Consent for Examination or Treatment* reinforces the importance of

47

The Department of Health's Response to the Report of the Public Inquiry into children's heart surgery at the Bristol Royal Infirmary 1984-1995

responding truthfully to patients' questions, be they adult or child. We have already acknowledged the importance of equipping health care professionals with the skills for good communication in this Response and set out proposals for doing this.

Health care services and treatment for children with congenital heart disease

Recommendations 192 - 198

Recommendation 192

National standards should be developed, as a matter of priority, for all aspects of the care and treatment of children with congenital heart disease (CHD). The standards should address diagnosis, surgical and other treatments, and continuing care. They should include standards for primary and social care, as well as for hospital care. The standards should also address the needs of those with CHD who grow into adulthood.

Recommendation 193

With regard to paediatric cardiac surgery, the standards should stipulate the minimum number of procedures which must be performed in a hospital over a given period of time in order to have the best opportunity of achieving good outcomes for children. PCS must not be undertaken in hospitals which do not meet the minimum number of procedures. Considerations of ease of access to a hospital should not be taken into account in determining whether PCS should be undertaken at that hospital.

Recommendation 194

With regard to those surgeons who undertake paediatric cardiac surgery, although not stipulating the number of operating sessions sufficient to maintain competence, it may be that four sessions a week should be the minimum number required. Agreement on this should be reached as a matter of urgency after appropriate consultation.

Recommendation 195

With regard to the very particular circumstances of open-heart surgery on very young children (including neo-nates and infants), we stipulate that the following standard should apply unless, within six months of the publication of this Report, this standard is varied by the DoH having taken the advice of relevant experts: there must, in any unit providing open-heart surgery on very young children, be two surgeons trained in paediatric surgery who must each undertake between 40 and 50 open-heart operations a year.

Recommendation 196

The national standards should stipulate that children with CHD who undergo any form of interventional procedure must be cared for in a paediatric environment. This means that all healthcare professionals who care for these children must be trained and qualified in paediatric care. It also means that children must be cared for in a setting with facilities and equipment designed for children. There must also be access on the same site where any surgery is performed to a paediatric intensive care unit, supported by trained intensivists.

Recommendation 197

Surgical services for children with very rare congenital heart conditions, such as Truncus Arteriosus, or involving procedures undertaken very rarely, should only be performed in a maximum of two units, validated as such on the advice of experts. Such arrangements should be subject to periodic review.

Recommendation 198

An investigation should be conducted as a matter of urgency to ensure that PCS is not currently being carried out where the low volume of patients or other factors make it unsafe to perform such surgery.

3.16   The arrangements for the care of children with congenital heart disease were the trigger for setting up the BRI Inquiry. It is right that services for these very sick young children should be accorded a particular focus as we move care forward, and plan how we will deliver highly specialised services for children in the future. Lessons have already been learnt by the NHS and the organisational arrangements, such as split site working and children being nursed in adult intensive care units, that pertained at Bristol until 1995 no longer apply there or elsewhere for children undergoing heart surgery.

3.17   The Kennedy Report makes a series of important recommendations about how paediatric services for children with congenital heart disease should be organised and managed in future. The Paediatric and Congenital Cardiac Services Review Group is looking specifically at these issues and will consider these recommendations. It is currently undertaking a thorough review of existing units providing paediatric cardiac surgery. We have asked it to make recommendations on the number of procedures to be undertaken by each unit and by each surgeon, and on the recommendation that very rare services should be undertaken by only two units. We expect the Group to report this year.

49

The Department of Health's Response to the Report of the Public Inquiry into children's heart surgery at the Bristol Royal Infirmary 1984-1995

3.18 In the meantime we are confident that real progress has been made over recent years in this specialist area of medicine. In 1985 over 1,200 children born with serious heart defects died. Today this figure is 75% lower. All paediatric cardiac surgery is carried out in specialist units with paediatric intensive care facilities on site. All the units participate in the Central Cardiac Audit Database (CCAD) and regularly review their clinical outcomes to ensure the services they provide are safe and of acceptable quality. In the case of Bristol all children's heart surgery is provided at the new Royal Bristol Children's Hospital which opened last year: its results are amongst the best in the country and its staff are to be commended on learning the lessons of Bristol.

3.19 Other initiatives in train for improving children's services include:

- clear standards for paediatric intensive care set out in *Paediatric Intensive Care: A Framework for the Future*, launched in July 1997;

- a strategy for neonatal intensive care for consultation later this year; and

- the development of good practice guidelines for paediatric high dependency care.

Conclusion

3.20 We recognise that we still have some way to go in providing the child-centred approach recommended by Professor Kennedy and his panel. The NSF and the Paediatric and Cardiac Congenital Services Review will take us some way to establishing clear standards and targets for the service: we are putting in place arrangements to give children's services a strong local focus; we will train staff and support parents in communicating with each other and we will encourage the greater integration of children's services so that unhelpful barriers between agencies and sectors are swept away. Through this multi-faceted approach we will move towards a service which is designed genuinely to reflect and meet the specific and particular needs of the children who use it.

3.21 In responding to the Kennedy Report's recommendations on the health care of children we will ensure that:

- there continues to be a high level focus for children's issues across government;

- every Strategic Health Authority, PCT and NHS Trust will have a senior member of staff with responsibility for children's services from April 2002;

- children's health services will be designed to meet the particular needs of the children who use them and their families. We will publish the NSF module on hospital care for children in 2002;

- the children's NSF will provide for greater integration of primary, community, acute and specialist health care across professional and agency boundaries;

- there will be clear standards against which providers of services are inspected as part of the Children's NSF;

- the Paediatric and Congenital Cardiac Services Review Group will make recommendations about the future configuration of paediatric cardiac services in 2002;

- all those operating on children will have had appropriate paediatric training; and

- parents will be fully engaged in decisions about their child's treatment and care.

Chapter 4

STANDARDS OF CARE

This chapter looks at how standards of care are set, promulgated and monitored to ensure that patients throughout the country have access to care and treatment which reflects the best available evidence. It also describes the systems for assessing performance locally and nationally and the arrangements for tackling under performance.

4.1   For most of the first 40 years of its existence, the National Health Service worked with an implicit notion of quality and standards of care. This built on the philosophy that well trained staff, good facilities and equipment automatically led to high standards. While medical and clinical audit was introduced in the 1980s and was widely undertaken across the NHS this was professionally led and dominated. The value to patients or the health service more generally was not apparent: health authorities decided levels and types of treatment and individual clinicians were answerable to their professional bodies for standards of care and the introduction of new treatments.

Our approach to standard setting

Recommendation 39

The framework of regulation must consist of two overarching organisations, independent of government, which bring together the various bodies which regulate healthcare. A Council for the Quality of Healthcare should be created to bring together those bodies which regulate healthcare standards and institutions (including, for example, the Commission for Health Improvement (CHI), the National Institute for Clinical Excellence (NICE) and the proposed National Patient Safety Agency). A Council for the Regulation of Healthcare Professionals should be created to bring together those bodies which regulate healthcare professionals (including, for example, the General Medical Council (GMC) and the Nursing and Midwifery Council); in effect, this is the body currently referred to in *'The NHS Plan'* as the Council of Healthcare Regulators. These overarching organisations must ensure that there is an integrated and co-ordinated approach to setting standards, monitoring performance, and inspection and validation. Issues of overlap and of gaps between the various bodies must be addressed and resolved.

Recommendation 40

The two Councils should be independent of government and report both to the DoH and to Parliament. There should be close collaboration between the two Councils. The DoH should establish and fund the Councils and set their strategic framework, and thereafter periodically review them.

Recommendation 41

The various bodies whose purpose it is to assure the quality of care in the NHS (for example, CHI and NICE) and the competence of healthcare professionals (for example, the GMC and the Nursing and Midwifery Council) must themselves be independent of and at arm's-length from the DoH.

Recommendation 42

All the various bodies and organisations concerned with regulation, besides being independent of government, must involve and reflect the interests of patients, the public and healthcare professionals, as well as the NHS and government.

4.2   The NHS White Paper *The New NHS* and the consultation paper *A First Class Service*, set out our strategy for ensuring more standard setting and quality management within the NHS. We agree with the proposals in the Kennedy Report that this framework should be made more explicit.

The Department of Health's Response to the Report of the Public Inquiry into children's heart surgery at the Bristol Royal Infirmary 1984-1995

4.3   Firstly, we agree with the view that those bodies set up to assure the quality of care in the NHS organisations – CHI, NICE, NCAA and NPSA - should work more closely together to establish a coherent approach to standard setting, regulation, monitoring and inspection of health care. We will establish a new Council for Quality of Health Care to help facilitate co-operative working between these constituent organisations; and help these bodies work closely together with the Social Services Inspectorate, the National Care Standards Commission, and the Audit Commission. The Council will help these organisations ensure that as far as possible methodologies, and timing of visits are aligned.

Figure 1:   The Framework for Quality

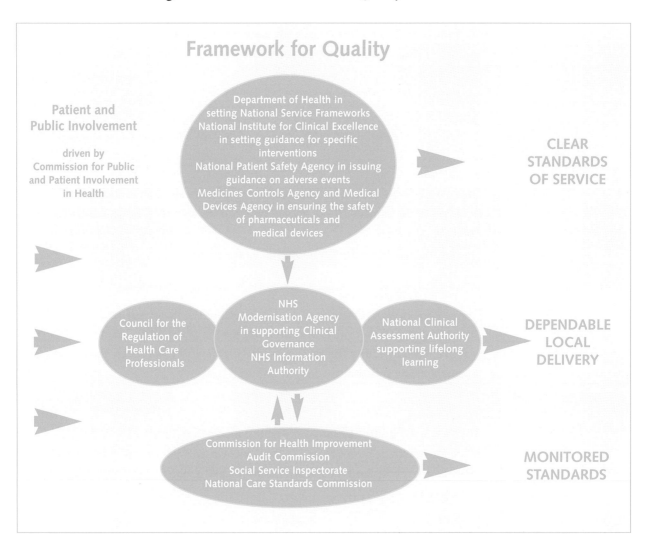

4.4   We have given careful thought to the view in the Kennedy Report that the various bodies whose purpose it is to assure the quality of care in the NHS should be independent of and at arm's length from the Department of Health. We endorse the view that they should be able to operate independently of the Department of Health in discharging their functions. We have signalled our intent significantly to strengthen the inspectorate process in the NHS Reform and Health Care Professions Bill. However, given the accountability of the Secretary of State to Parliament we believe that the proper role of these bodies should be to operate within a framework of priorities set by government against the overall resourcing of the NHS.

4.5   These bodies are still very new and developing ways of working with the NHS. We wish to minimise the disruption caused by the establishment of new bodies or changes in the existing bodies. For these reasons we have decided to leave their existing accountability intact. CHI will continue to be a non departmental public body, independent of and at arm's length from the Department of Health, but will in future provide an annual report to Parliament on its findings on the quality of the NHS. NICE and NPSA will continue as Special Health Authorities, with a clear framework of priorities set by the Secretary of State but with greater independence to implement them.

Setting standards

4.6   The Kennedy Report describes the confusion in the past about which standards should apply within the NHS. We have repeatedly set out our commitment to providing fair access to services and high standards of care for patients wherever they live. National standards are now being developed through:

- **The National Institute for Clinical Excellence**, which produces clear guidance on clinically and cost effective health care. It has to date issued 4 sets of clinical guidelines with 31 more clinical and service guidelines in its work programme, and 31 sets of technology appraisal guidance with a further 44 in its work programme.

- **National Service Frameworks** setting national standards for key conditions and diseases. NSFs have already been issued for coronary heart disease, mental health and older people and the *National Cancer Plan* was published in September 2000. NSFs are in preparation for diabetes, renal services, children and long-term conditions.

- **The Performance Assessment Framework** and clear national targets. The Framework helps to assess the performance of the NHS in health improvement; fair access; effective delivery of appropriate care; efficiency; patient/carer experience and health outcomes of NHS care.

Authoritative clinical standards

Recommendations 122 - 129

Recommendation 122

One body should be responsible for co-ordinating *all* action relating to the setting, issuing and keeping under review of national clinical standards: this should be NICE, suitably structured so as to give it the necessary independence and authority.

Recommendation 123

Once the recommended system is in place, only NICE should be permitted to issue national clinical standards to the NHS. The DoH (as the headquarters of the NHS) while issuing, for example, National Service Frameworks and supplementary guidance, should not be able to rescind or detract from the standards issued by NICE.

Recommendation 124

NICE should pursue vigorously its current policy of involving as wide a community as possible, including the public, patients and carers, in the work to develop and keep under review clinical standards. In particular, the special expertise of the Royal Colleges and specialist professional associations should be harnessed and supported. Account should also be taken of the expertise of the senior management of the NHS.

Recommendation 125

National standards of clinical care should reflect the commitment to patient-centred care and thus in future be formulated from the perspective of the patient. The standards should address the quality of care that a patient with a given illness or condition is entitled to expect to receive from the NHS. The standards should take account of the best available evidence. The standards should include guidance on how promptly patients should get access to care. They should address the roles and responsibilities of the various healthcare professionals who will care for the patient. They should take account of the patient's journey from primary care, into the hospital system (if necessary), and back to primary and community care, and of the necessary facilities and equipment.

> **Recommendation 126**
>
> Such standards for clinical care as are established should distinguish clearly between those which are obligatory and must be observed, and those to which the NHS should aspire over time.
>
> **Recommendation 127**
>
> A timetable over the short, medium and long term should be published, and revised periodically, for the development of national clinical standards, so that the public may be consulted and kept aware of those areas of healthcare which are covered by such standards and those which will be covered in the future. Target dates should be set by which clinical standards will have been prepared for all major conditions and illnesses.
>
> **Recommendation 128**
>
> Resources, and any necessary statutory authority, must be made available to NICE to allow it to perform its role of developing, issuing and keeping under review national clinical standards.
>
> **Recommendation 129**
>
> Standards of clinical care which patients are entitled to expect to receive in the NHS should be made public.

4.7   Since April 1999 NICE has been the foremost body charged with providing authoritative guidance to the NHS in the form of clinical guidelines and technology appraisals. NICE advice is already independent of any vested interests. As a Special Health Authority NICE can operate at arm's length from government while being part of the NHS. We believe that it is this relationship with the NHS that gives it authority and credibility with those who must implement its recommendations.

4.8   However, although NICE currently operates with considerable independence - critically itself determining the standards it sets - we consider that this could be further strengthened by:

- removing the requirement for approval from the Secretary of State for Health and the National Assembly for Wales for disseminating NICE guidance; and

- enabling NICE to determine its own committee structure and to appoint members to committees without reference to the Secretary of State or the National Assembly for Wales.

57

The Department of Health's Response to the Report of the Public Inquiry into children's heart surgery at the Bristol Royal Infirmary 1984-1995

4.9   In line with the recommendations in the Kennedy report, we will also sharpen NICE's focus as the main standard setting body for the NHS. It already is responsible for setting authoritative standards of clinical practice through its guidelines and technology appraisals. NICE guidance will also provide the clinical core for National Service Frameworks. These also provide important information to patients as they set out the kind of clinical service and treatment which patients can expect.

4.10   NICE will also take over responsibility for the Safety and Efficacy Register of New Interventional Procedures (SERNIP) which considers and categorises new surgical treatments according to their safety and efficacy. Where safety and efficacy have not been established, treatments should only be provided as part of a clinical trial until these have been put beyond doubt. The Government is also giving serious consideration to NICE taking on responsibility for advice to the NHS on clinical standards for screening interventions. Furthermore, the Government is considering whether there are other forms of guidance which are currently developed outside of NICE, but which might more appropriately fall within NICE's remit.

4.11   These changes will make NICE the pre-eminent authority in setting clinical standards. It cannot be the **only** setter of standards. Bodies such as the Medicines Control Agency, the Medical Devices Agency and the National Patient Safety Agency will continue to have clear responsibility for standards in their own fields. The Royal Colleges and professional associations also provide guidance to their members. Where NICE guidance exists it provides the standard. Advice from professional bodies which goes beyond NICE guidance may be regarded as aspirational and will provide an incentive to improve practice. Where there are conflicts, NICE guidance must be paramount.

4.12   The Government recognises that a number of concerns have been put forward about the current process for identifying and selecting topics for appraisal by NICE. We are therefore publishing a consultation document covering the detail of the process of topic selection.

4.13   The guidance produced by NICE will continue to be evidence based and carefully prepared through six National Collaborating Centres based in the Royal Colleges for clinical guidelines and through an Appraisal Committee for technology appraisals. Patient groups will continue to be helped to participate in the development of NICE guidance. The influence of patients and the public in NICE guidance will be further advanced by the establishment of the Citizens' Council. NICE guidance will continue to be published.

4.14 The Government is fully committed to the work of NICE. We expect the NHS and health care professionals to take full and proper account of NICE guidance when it is issued. In order further to strengthen this we have introduced a statutory duty on NHS bodies to ensure that funding is available to support the provision of drugs and treatments recommended by NICE. This will be a major step in ensuring that recommended treatments are indeed provided. We will also ensure that sufficient resources are available to the NHS to enable this to be implemented.

4.15 To enable NICE to do its work effectively, we shall be further increasing its own resources to enable it to meet the commitments set out here and in *The NHS Plan.*

Generic standards

> **Recommendation 130**
>
> **There must be a single, coherent, co-ordinated set of generic standards: that is, standards relating to the patient's experience and the systems for ensuring that care is safe and of good quality (for example corporate management, clinical governance, risk management, clinical audit, the management and support of staff, and the management of resources). Trusts must comply with these standards.**

4.16 We agree that there must be a coherent underpinning for judging how well NHS Trusts ensure good quality, safe care and provide care in an environment of an appropriate standard. Clinical governance places upon organisations a clear responsibility for the delivery and continuous improvement of patient care – it is the mechanism for ensuring local delivery of national standards, local ownership for modernising patient care and also the process by which NHS organisations can demonstrate that they are meeting the statutory duty of quality set out in the Health Act 1999.

4.17 Clinical governance already provides a comprehensive framework against which to judge an organisation's ability to deliver continuous improvement in the quality of its services and standards of provision. It is this framework which CHI's clinical governance reviews assess. Clinical governance is being given strong support throughout the NHS by the National Clinical Governance Support Team (CGST), part of the NHS Modernisation Agency.

4.18   Already 276 teams in 232 organisations have attended the Clinical Governance Development Programme which provides health care staff with the opportunity to take a fresh look at the way in which they and their organisations deliver patient care. 36 NHS Trust boards have also been through a specially designed NHS Trust board programme.

4.19   The governance of a health care organisation has two prime components – corporate governance and clinical governance. In line with HM Treasury requirements, all NHS organisations must maintain effective systems of internal control, covering financial, organisational and clinical controls. A 'Statement on Internal Control' must be signed off by the Chief Executive on behalf of the NHS Trust board, in the Annual Report. The Department of Health is clarifying these requirements so that NHS Trust boards are clearer about their responsibilities for the quality of services and care delivered by their NHS Trusts, and the governance arrangements which need to be in place, with further guidance to be issued shortly.

Performance assessments, the inspection of NHS Trusts and validation

Recommendations 131 - 141

Recommendation 131
The current system of inspection of trusts and primary care trusts should be changed to become a system of validation and periodic revalidation of these trusts. The system should be supportive and flexible. Its aim should be to promote continued improvement in the quality of care.

Recommendation 132
One body should be responsible for validating and re-validating NHS trusts and primary care trusts. This body should be CHI, suitably structured so as to give it the necessary independence and authority. Other bodies (for example the NHS Litigation Authority) which are currently concerned with setting and requiring compliance with those generic standards which should fall within the authority of CHI, should carry out their role in this respect under the authority of and answerable to CHI.

Recommendation 133
Validation and revalidation of trusts should be based upon compliance with the generic standards which relate to the patient's experience and the systems for ensuring that care is safe and of good quality.

Recommendation 134

The standards against which trusts are to be validated, and the results of the process of validation or revalidation, should be made public.

Recommendation 135

Any organisation in the voluntary or private sector which provides services to NHS patients should be required to meet the standards for systems, facilities and staff which organisations in the NHS must meet. The aim should be that, wherever care is funded by the NHS, there is a single system of validation which indicates to the public that the organisation meets the necessary standards.

Recommendation 136

The validating body should have the power to withdraw, withhold or suspend a trust's validation if standards fall such as to threaten the quality of care or the safety of patients. Any trust or organisation whose validation may be affected in this way must be given the opportunity to take appropriate remedial action. It must then satisfy CHI that it has taken remedial action before its continued validation can be confirmed.

Recommendation 137

CHI should consider how it might work with the providers of those programmes of accreditation already adopted by a significant number of trusts. In the future, where required standards are met, CHI should accept as part of its validation process the accreditation obtained through these programmes.

Recommendation 138

The process of validation of trusts should, in time, be extended to cover discrete, identifiable services within trusts. This extension of validation should first be piloted and evaluated.

Recommendation 139

The pilot exercise for this form of validation should include children's acute hospital services and paediatric cardiac surgery.

Recommendation 140

Should the pilot exercise be successful, the category of discrete services which should be a priority for this form of validation are those specialist services which are currently funded or meet the criteria for funding by the National Specialist Commissioning Group (the successor to the Supra Regional Services Advisory Group).

> **Recommendation 141**
>
> **For discrete services, whether specialist services or otherwise, to be validated trusts they must be able to demonstrate that all relevant aspects of the service can *currently* be met, rather than that the trust *aims* to develop so as to be able to do so at some point in the future. Trusts which do not meet the necessary standards to ensure the safety of patients and a good quality of care should not be permitted to offer, or continue to offer, the relevant service.**

4.20 Establishing a clearer framework of standards is not enough. We believe that there should be a strong mechanism for assessing performance against these standards and that it should be at arm's length from the Department of Health. To this end, the role of CHI will be strengthened in the NHS Reform and Health Care Professions Bill. In future CHI will have a new function of inspecting individual NHS Trusts and other service providers offering NHS care in line with specified criteria. These criteria will be derived from NSFs, NICE guidelines, the Controls Assurance framework and guidance from the Department of Health and the Royal Colleges. The criteria, which will be set in agreement with the Secretary of State for Health will cover:

- clinical services;

- services related to the patient;

- environment;

- safety and quality ; and

- financial and management performance.

These criteria will be made public.

4.21 We have given careful thought to the system of validation and revalidation of NHS Trusts as recommended by the Kennedy Report but must reject this proposal. The Secretary of State for Health has a statutory duty for the provision of health services. Giving CHI the role of withdrawing an NHS Trust's validation and effectively requiring it to stop offering some or all of its services, without consideration of alternative provision, could have a major and detrimental impact on the delivery of services to sectors of the population. It could lead to a loss of NHS capacity at a time when the Government is seeking to expand it in order to offer more patients more high quality treatment more quickly.

4.22 We do however take seriously the need to act swiftly where there are major problems or where patient safety is compromised. We therefore propose, through the NHS Reform and Health Care Professions Bill, to give CHI the power and the responsibility to recommend 'special measures' for NHS Trusts which are failing to meet the required standards.

4.23 Following an inspection, CHI would be under a duty to report to the Secretary of State that - on the basis of the inspection report or analysis of data from the NHS Trust - they believe the health care for which the body is responsible is of unacceptably poor quality or there are significant failings in the way it is being run. This judgement would apply to standards of care generally throughout an NHS Trust or to discrete services. The Secretary of State would then decide what action to take including special measures such as:

- re-inspection by CHI within a certain period;

- action by the NHS Modernisation Agency to assist the body in improving the quality of its health care;

- the use of intervention powers such as those currently provided in section 84A of the 1977 NHS Act;

- suspension or alternative arrangements for the provision of a clinical service; or

- franchising of the management or services of the NHS Trust.

4.24 In this way there would be an immediate and effective response to identified concerns about an NHS Trust's performance taken within the context of ensuring alternative provision for the affected population. Professor Kennedy expresses concern that there is potential for inconsistency and fragmentation whilst a number of bodies retain responsibility for inspection and recommends some rationalisation and a reappraisal of the future role of the Audit Commission in addressing issues to do with clinical effectiveness and the comparative performance of NHS bodies. We accept the logic of this and will take further steps at the earliest opportunity. In the meantime CHI will work more closely with other inspecting and accrediting bodies, particularly the National Care Standards Commission and the Social Services Inspectorate. We will make provision in the NHS Reform and Health Care Professions Bill for the Audit Commission to consult CHI on its relevant programmes of work in relation to the health service. We will begin to move away from the fragmentation that Professor Kennedy has highlighted, towards a more integrated approach to the inspection of all those who provide care for NHS patients.

The role of the Office for Information on Health Care Performance

Recommendations 146, 147

Recommendation 146

The monitoring of clinical performance at a national level should be brought together and co-ordinated in one body: an independent Office for Information on Healthcare Performance. This Office should be part of CHI.

Recommendation 147

The Office for Information on Healthcare Performance should supplant the current fragmentation of approach through a programme of activities involving the co-ordination of the various national audits. In addition to its other responsibilities, the new system should provide a mechanism for surveillance whereby patterns of performance in the NHS which may warrant further scrutiny can be identified as early as possible.

4.25 The Government has already announced its intention to establish an Office for Information on Health Care Performance as part of CHI to monitor clinical performance at national level. The Office for Information on Health Care Performance would:

- bring together data from a variety of existing and future data collection systems including that collected by the Department of Health - to carry out routine surveillance and underpin early identification of potential problems;

- analyse that data to identify good and bad performance, and act as a prompt to CHI's service inspections;

- publish reports with selected data and analysis, including NHS performance ratings;

- assess the adequacy of current data used to describe the quality and performance of the NHS, evaluate the systems for data collection and analysis and make recommendations for improving them;

- co-ordinate systems for the collection of data from clinical audit;

- commission national audits ; and

- carry out national patient and staff surveys and publish the results.

4.26 In this way:

- standards of care will be put at the heart of NHS performance assessment;

- improvements in the performance of the NHS will be independently verifiable and presented publicly;

- the culture of the NHS will be changed so that routinely collected data are seen as relevant to clinical practice, the quality of data becomes reliable and the wasteful dual collection of administrative and clinical data can be ended;

- indicators used to assess clinical performance will be developed which are seen as useful by clinicians in helping them improve performance;

- information will be reported that is relevant to what patients and the public want and ought to know;

- up to date information will be available for the assessment of NHS performance ; and

- the system of standards, inspection and performance assessment will be coherent and co-ordinated.

4.27 We propose that the Office for Information on Health Care Performance will be responsible for taking forward the work on performance indicators for all NHS activity, with parameters set by the Department of Health. We have, however, decided not to transfer responsibility for the National Confidential Enquiries to CHI. For the time being they will remain with NICE. The fundamental role of the Enquiries is to gather information on post-operative deaths, maternal deaths and stillbirths, deaths in infancy, and suicides and homicides by people with mental illness to enable lessons to be learned and good practice promulgated. Their methodologies are not set up as an audit tool, nor a service by service comparison of performance. They are a way of identifying trends in avoidable factors in deaths and enabling professional practice and NHS policies to respond to prevent future deaths.

65

The Department of Health's Response to the Report of the Public Inquiry into children's heart surgery at the Bristol Royal Infirmary 1984-1995

4.28 CHI will remain a non departmental public body. This puts it at arm's length from government. To reinforce its independence of government, the Director of Health Improvement will be appointed by the Commission itself, without the need for the agreement of the Secretary of State, and CHI will be required to complete an annual report on the quality of NHS services, to be laid before Parliament. This will detail:

- the quality of NHS health care; and

- the success of NHS organisations in developing clinical governance arrangements for assuring, monitoring and improving the quality of health care.

4.29 The Kennedy Report recommended that priority should be given to validating those specialist services currently funded by the National Specialist Commissioning Advisory Group (NSCAG). NSCAG exists to ensure the highest possible standard of care that can be delivered within available resources is available to all NHS patients requiring treatment or investigation of a very specialised nature, or for a very uncommon condition. Whilst not accepting validation for those services we recognise that they should only be delivered in a small number of centres and we accept that quality and safety should be the prevailing criteria. NSCAG services are subject to the same external scrutiny as any other services – including cross-cutting inspections by CHI, underpinned by robust inter-unit audit and, increasingly, by the development of national standards against which they can be assessed. This will always be at the heart of any future reconfiguration of health service facilities.

Conclusion

4.30 If we are to continue to drive forward the impetus for improved quality across the NHS as a whole we need to be clear about the standards that are in place and have an effective and independent system of performance assessment against those standards. For this reason we are strengthening the roles of NICE and CHI, establishing the Office for Information on Health Care Performance and developing standards which will form the core of regular CHI inspections along with their inspection of the local NHS organisation's quality assurance and improvement (i.e. clinical governance arrangements). CHI will submit an annual report on the quality of NHS services which the Secretary of State will lay before Parliament.

4.31 Shortfalls or weaknesses in the service may be identified through those external processes or the Department of Health's own collection of information and performance management arrangements. Performance management solutions will themselves be tested again as part of performance assessment: in this way our actions and those of the NHS will continue to be subject to ongoing independent scrutiny as an important element in the drive to deliver high quality and safe patient care.

4.32 We will take the following action, through legislation where necessary, in response to the Kennedy Report's recommendations on setting the standards of care:

- clear standards will be set through NICE and the NSFs;

- the independence of CHI will be reinforced in the NHS Reform and Health Care Professions Bill;

- NHS bodies will be directed to fund treatments recommended by NICE;

- NICE guidance will no longer need to be approved by the Secretary of State for Health before dissemination;

- CHI will be strengthened to take on the role of inspection of NHS organisations and service providers against a new and additional set of core standards for the NHS;

- swift action will be taken where CHI identifies significant problems or where patient safety is compromised, including the imposition of 'special measures';

- the Office for Information on Health Care Performance will be established as part of CHI to monitor clinical performance;

- the Office for Information on Health Care Performance will publish regular performance indicators for all NHS Trusts and PCTs; and

- CHI will appoint its own Director of Health Improvement and will produce an annual report on the quality of NHS services which the Secretary of State will lay before Parliament.

Chapter 5

THE SAFETY OF CARE

This chapter outlines work in hand to establish a system for analysing and learning from adverse events throughout the NHS and developing the NHS as a learning organisation, with the aim of reducing harm to patients caused through error.

5.1 The Kennedy Report found that the NHS is still failing to learn from things that go wrong and that the prevailing blame culture is a major barrier to openness and learning. Patient safety is at the centre of our agenda for improving the quality of NHS services and is becoming a key priority for health services around the world. As such, it is a key responsibility for NHS Trust boards and PCTs collectively as part of clinical governance. *An Organisation with a Memory* published in July 2000, was a turning point. For the first time in 50 years, attention was drawn to the scale of unintended harm to patients from potentially avoidable error in the health care system:

- adverse events occur in around 10% of admissions (equal to 850,000 adverse events a year);

- 400 people die or are seriously injured in adverse events involving medical devices every year;

- additional hospital stays as a result of adverse effects; and

- settlement of clinical negligence claims of around £400 million a year.

A single national system of reporting adverse events

Recommendations 106 - 112

Recommendation 106

We support and endorse the broad framework of recommendations advocated in the report *'An Organisation with a Memory'* by the Chief Medical Officer's expert group on learning from adverse events in the NHS. The National Patient Safety Agency proposed as a consequence of that report should, like all other bodies which contribute to the regulation of the safety and quality of healthcare, be independent of the NHS and the DoH.

Recommendation 107

Every effort should be made to create in the NHS an open and non-punitive environment in which it is safe to report and admit sentinel events.

Recommendation 108

Major studies should, as a matter of priority, be carried out to investigate the extent and type of sentinel events in the NHS to establish a baseline against which improvements can be made and measured.

Recommendation 109

There should a single, unified, accessible system for reporting and analysing sentinel events, with clear protocols indicating the categories of information which must be reported to a national database.

Recommendation 110

The national database of sentinel events should be managed by the National Patient Safety Agency, so as to ensure that a high degree of confidence is placed in the system by the public.

Recommendation 111

The National Patient Safety Agency, in the exercise of its function of surveillance of sentinel events, should be required to inform all trusts of the need for immediate action, in the light of occurrences reported to it. The Agency should also be required to publish regular reports on patterns of sentinel events and proposed remedial actions.

Recommendation 112

All sentinel events should be subject to a form of structured analysis in the trust where they occur, which takes into account not only the conduct of individuals, but also the wider contributing factors within the organisation which may have given rise to the event.

69

The Department of Health's Response to the Report of the Public Inquiry into children's heart surgery at the Bristol Royal Infirmary 1984-1995

5.2 The Kennedy Report recommends a single unified and accessible system for reporting and analysing sentinel events with clear protocols indicating which categories of information must be reported to a national database. This was the view set out in *An Organisation with a Memory*. We are grateful to Professor Kennedy for reviewing experience on patient safety world-wide and endorsing the philosophy and approach as set out in *An Organisation with a Memory*. The Government set out its plans to implement this Report and improve patient safety in *Building a Safer NHS for Patients*. A central commitment was the establishment of the National Patient Safety Agency with the following remit:

- to devise and implement a reporting system based on relevant national standards issued by the Department of Health regarding adverse incidents;

- to collect and appraise information on reported adverse incidents and other material useful for any purpose connected with the promotion of patient safety;

- to provide advice and guidance useful in the maintenance and promotion of patient safety and to monitor the effectiveness of such advice and guidance;

- to promote research which the Agency considers will contribute to improvements in patient safety ; and

- to report to and advise Ministers on matters affecting patient safety.

5.3 The NPSA was established in July 2001 as a Special Health Authority to work at arm's length from the Department of Health and discussions are underway with the National Assembly for Wales and the Scottish Parliament about extending the NPSA's remit to those countries. The Agency has one core purpose - to improve patient safety by reducing the risk of harm through error. Its work has already started.

5.4 We consider that its status as a Special Health Authority provides the independence necessary to give the Agency credibility with patients and carers while its place within the NHS 'family' enables it to command the confidence of health care staff, to work with stakeholders in related fields and to ensure that its recommendations for improving practice are credible and acted on.

5.5   In line with the blueprint outlined in *Building a Safer NHS for Patients*, a national system for reporting and analysing adverse events and 'near misses' is being piloted in 28 NHS Trusts and will be evaluated prior to national roll out in 2002. Draft guidance on the proposed reporting arrangements, currently entitled *Doing Less Harm,* has been prepared for the pilot sites, and is available at www.npsa.org.uk .

5.6   The Kennedy Report suggests that the term 'sentinel event' should be used for those events which are to be reported - meaning any unexplained occurrence involving death or serious physical or psychological injury, or risk thereof. The definition of an 'adverse event' in the NPSA's current draft guidance is 'any event or circumstance arising during NHS care that could have or did lead to unexpected harm, loss or damage'.

5.7   'Harm' is defined as 'injury (physical or psychological), disease, suffering, disability or death'. In most cases, harm can be considered to be 'unexpected' if it is not related to the natural cause of the patient's illness or underlying condition. The NPSA is testing these definitions in the piloting work.

5.8   The experience gained from the pilots and the early stages of the operation of the national system together with analyses in hand of existing databases will provide baseline data against which to measure future improvements, as the Kennedy Report proposes.

5.9   The database of reported events will be managed by the NPSA which will analyse the data collected from NHS organisations, staff, patients and carers alongside safety information from other sources in this country and abroad. From these analyses, lessons will be learned and fed back, as quickly as possible to relevant stakeholders in the NHS and elsewhere. In this way, organisations and individual clinicians and managers will be able to change practice to reduce the risk for future patients and to improve the safety and quality of patient care.

5.10   At the local level, NHS staff and organisations will be encouraged to learn the lessons from adverse events by investigating the 'root causes' – rather than simply seeking to allocate blame. Guidance on root cause analysis has been developed and will form part of the roll out programme of the new reporting system. The guidance describes how local NHS Trusts can undertake a structured analysis of adverse events or near misses, including the human and other factors most directly associated with the event and the process and systems related to its occurrence.

Incentives to encourage reporting

Recommendations 113 - 118

Recommendation 113

The reporting of sentinel events must be made as easy as possible, using all available means of communication (including a confidential telephone reporting line).

Recommendation 114

Members of staff in the NHS should receive immunity from disciplinary action by the employer or by a professional body if they report a sentinel event to the trust or to the national database within 48 hours, except where they themselves have committed a criminal offence.

Recommendation 115

Members of staff in the NHS who cover up or do not report a sentinel event may be subject to disciplinary action by their employer or by their professional body.

Recommendation 116

The opportunity should exist to report a sentinel event in confidence.

Recommendation 117

There should be a stipulation in every healthcare professional's contract that sentinel events must be reported, that reporting can be confidential, and that reporting within a specified time period will not attract disciplinary action.

Recommendation 118

The process of reporting of sentinel events should be integrated into every trust's internal communications, induction training and other staff training. Staff must know what is expected of them, to whom to report and what systems are in place to enable them to report.

5.11 The core purpose of the reporting system being established by the NPSA is to learn from events which harm, or have the capacity to cause harm to patients so that changes in care practices can be identified and introduced and patient safety improved. This learning will take place locally (i.e. within the NHS organisation) and nationally. International links are also being forged.

5.12 The success of the reporting system will, as the Kennedy report recognises, depend crucially on developing a reporting and a safety culture in local NHS organisations. The challenge of this should not be underestimated. The NPSA will be looking for mechanisms to ensure the confidentiality of reporting. It will require a massive commitment from organisations and staff for the NHS itself to become an organisation which learns from things which go wrong both locally and more widely. The need to become a learning organisation and to change from the current blame culture is well recognised. To this end training will be provided for all staff so they know what they are expected to report and to whom within their organisation. There will also be the facility for staff (and patients and carers) to report direct to the NPSA. We see merit in principle in the recommendation to introduce a requirement in staff contracts to report adverse events - with immunity from disciplinary action for reporting within 48 hours of the event but disciplinary action for failing to report an adverse event. We will bring forward detailed proposals in the White Paper on Clinical Negligence to be published early in 2002. Immunity would not apply if a criminal offence was committed.

Additional patient safety initiatives

Recommendations 120, 121

Recommendation 120

The proposed National Patient Safety Agency should, as a matter of urgency, bring together managers in the NHS, representatives of the pharmaceutical companies and manufacturers of medical equipment, members of the healthcare professions and the public, to seek to apply approaches based on engineering and design so as to reduce (and eliminate to the extent possible) the incidence of sentinel events.

Recommendation 121

At the level of individual trusts, an executive member of the board should have the responsibility for putting into operation the trust's strategy and policy on safety in clinical care. Further, a non-executive director should be given specific responsibility for providing leadership to the strategy and policy aimed at securing safety in clinical care.

5.13 The comprehensive approach outlined in *Building a Safer NHS for Patients* identifies the need to:

- review the safety environment;

- review clinical practice;

- consider the scope for safety briefings;

- harness the potential of new technologies through the use of computers to reduce error and simulate risk in special laboratories;

- explore the potential for patients to play a role in promoting safety;

- purchase for safety; and

- design for safety, which the Kennedy Report particularly highlights.

5.14 Action in hand includes:

- the development of guidance with the Purchasing and Supplies Authority for local NHS procurement staff on purchasing for safety;

- working with the Design Council to bring together key players to identify a range of areas where design can play its part in enhancing safety, in particular to reduce medication error and errors in obstetrics and gynaecology;

- the Medicines Control Agency's recent consultation on changes in the packaging and labelling of medicines to improve safety; and

- a trial to assess the simulation training and team safety briefing in labour wards.

5.15 Professor Kennedy recommends that an executive member of the board should have responsibility for putting into operation a Trust's strategy for clinical safety and that a non-executive should be designated to give leadership. We believe clinical safety is of such critical importance that it should be a collective responsibility of the entire board. But we do recognise that NHS Trust and PCT boards may need help in meeting their clinical safety responsibilities and that a non-executive should be designated to provide leadership.

5.16 Following the publication of the Kennedy Report and noting the importance that was placed on the role of the non-executive directors of NHS boards in patient safety, the Chief Medical Officer jointly with the NPSA and the NHS Confederation has held a series of 'roadshows' for non-executive directors in all parts of the country. This has familiarised board members with the subject of patient safety; set out the philosophy of 'safe systems'; and described the action being taken in the NHS. Their crucial role was addressed in a series of ten key questions that they were asked to use to challenge their own organisations.

- Are patient safety and clinical governance key objectives for the organisation and considered by the board?

- Do induction and development programmes include patient safety issues?

- What is being done to educate/inform the workforce about patient safety issues?

- Can you demonstrate indisputably that your service is becoming safer to patients year in year out?

- Can the management and clinical teams show you examples of where through analysing something that has gone wrong, care of future patients will be much safer?

- Is your organisation in regular contact or twinned with another organisation in a different sector in the UK or in health care internationally which has a reputation for excellence in safety?

- What is your organisation doing to reduce the risk of medication error (which accounts for a quarter of all harm to patients)?

- Pick the worst three errors you have heard of and ask managers and professional staff if they could happen in your organisation.

- If something serious happened would the culture of your organisation be to cover it up or learn from it?

- Are patients actively involved in activities to improve safety and reduce risk?

75

The Department of Health's Response to the Report of the Public Inquiry into children's heart surgery at the Bristol Royal Infirmary 1984-1995

The acquisition and development of new clinical skills

> ### Recommendations 99 - 103
>
> #### Recommendation 99
>
> **Any clinician carrying out any clinical procedure for the first time must be directly supervised by colleagues who have the necessary skill, competence and experience until such time as the relevant degree of expertise has been acquired.**
>
> #### Recommendation 100
>
> **Before any *new* and hitherto untried invasive clinical procedure can be undertaken for the first time, the clinician involved should have to satisfy the relevant local research ethics committee that the procedure is justified and it is in the patient's interests to proceed. Each trust should have in place a system for ensuring that this process is complied with.**
>
> #### Recommendation 101
>
> **Local research ethics committees should be re-formed as necessary so that they are capable of considering applications to undertake new and hitherto untried invasive clinical procedures.**
>
> #### Recommendation 102
>
> **Patients are always entitled to know the extent to which a procedure which they are about to undergo is innovative or experimental. They are also entitled to be informed about the experience of the clinician who is to carry out the procedure.**
>
> #### Recommendation 103
>
> **The Royal College of Surgeons of England should, in partnership with university medical schools and the NHS, be enabled to develop its unit for the training of surgeons, particularly in new techniques. It should also explore the question of whether there is an age beyond which surgeons, specifically in areas such as paediatric cardiac surgery, should not attempt new procedures or even should not continue in a particular field of surgery.**

5.17 Having a national reporting system for adverse events is important, but we must also do what we can to minimise the number of adverse events occurring. We are fully committed to improving the quality of clinical care and have demonstrated this through *A First Class Service, The NHS Plan* and the establishment of NICE and CHI. A key area of concern identified in the Kennedy Report is when clinicians carry out clinical procedures for the first time.

5.18 Consultant clinicians are responsible for providing support for and ensuring the direct supervision of the members of their team, when taking on procedures that are new to them. They must themselves have undergone the appropriate education, training and supervision for the procedure in question. We recognise that though this is generally the case, the position should be formalised and reinforced through personal accountability and clinical governance. We are therefore working with the BMA on developing job plans for consultants, which will include specific accountability arrangements and supervision responsibilities in relation to themselves and their trainees, non-consultant staff and locums. We will issue further guidance on supervision as part of clinical governance responsibilities and it will be covered in the new annual appraisals and revalidation programmes. It is also part of the current and developing trainee assessment programmes.

5.19 But in addition to these arrangements we believe that the introduction of new interventional procedures needs special oversight and scrutiny. Given the need for detailed and scarce expert knowledge in the proper evaluation of the safety and efficacy of new interventions we believe this is a role best undertaken at national level. As already indicated in paragraph 4.10 we have asked NICE to take on responsibility for the Safety and Efficacy Register of New Interventional Procedures (SERNIP) from April 2002 rather than place responsibility with local research ethics committees as the Kennedy Report suggests. Ethical expertise will of course be needed within the new system and we will discuss cross-membership with research ethics committees to ensure good governance.

5.20 We will issue guidance on the new arrangements in 2002, including the responsibilities of individual clinicians and the organisations in which they work in relation to new interventional procedures. This will specify the local systems, which NHS Trusts will need to have in place for managing new interventional procedures as part of clinical governance.

5.21 In line with our view that there should be greater openness in health care we fully endorse the Inquiry's recommendation that patients should be told when the treatment being offered is of an experimental nature. Our *Reference Guide to Consent for Examination or Treatment* makes it clear that patients should be fully informed about experimental procedures, the degree of effectiveness and the practitioner's own experience, and given information about standard alternatives so that they can reach an informed choice.

5.22 The training of surgeons in new techniques is an essential component in the introduction of new procedures. We have provided significant support for the development of the Royal College of Surgeons of England's training unit for surgeons, especially in new techniques and simulator training. We will work with the College and NICE on the training requirements for any new interventional procedures they recommend.

5.23 The Kennedy Report suggests that the question should be considered of whether there is an age beyond which surgeons (and specifically paediatric cardiac surgeons) should not attempt new procedures or even continue in a particular field of surgery. There are already accepted rules about chronological age and clinicians continuing to work in the context of retirement, and for those who are retired in certain disciplines. We have already asked the Paediatric and Congenital Cardiac Services Review Group to look at the clinician age for paediatric cardiac surgery and we will consider doing this for other specialties. However, we believe that monitoring performance through audit in which all doctors must take part, the annual appraisal process and revalidation will help inform decisions on the scope of an individual clinician's practice.

5.24 One of the ways in future of addressing skill training, retraining, assessment and safer care, will undoubtedly be through the development of clinical skills centres and laboratories. It seems surprising that until relatively recently, all staff in training undertook their first procedure on an actual patient. Increasingly medical and nursing students are learning to put up drips, give injections and insert catheters on realistic mannequins. They hone their skills before having to treat patients. This can only lead to safer care and be better for the confidence of both patients and staff. Already there are simulated operating theatres where theatre teams can be trained in managing critical incidents. Many will never have dealt with one in real life but will be prepared when they do so in future. In the past, preparation for clinical crisis management has been patchy. These types of simulation centres will have a greatly expanded role in the future.

The system of clinical negligence

> ### Recommendations 33, 34, 37, 119
>
> #### Recommendation 33
> **A duty of candour, meaning a duty to tell a patient if adverse events have occurred, must be recognised as owed by all those working in the NHS to patients.**
>
> #### Recommendation 34
> **When things go wrong, patients are entitled to receive an acknowledgement, an explanation and an apology.**
>
> #### Recommendation 37
> **There should be an urgent review of the system for providing compensation to those who suffer harm arising out of medical care. The review should be concerned with the introduction of an administrative system for responding promptly to patients' needs in place of the current system of clinical negligence and should take account of other administrative systems for meeting the financial needs of the public.**
>
> #### Recommendation 119
> **In order to remove the disincentive to open reporting and the discussion of sentinel events represented by the clinical negligence system, this system should be abolished. It should be replaced by an alternative system for compensating those patients who suffer harm arising out of treatment from the NHS. An expert group should be established to advise on the appropriate method of compensation to be adopted.**

5.25 The current system for dealing with clinical negligence claims is recognised as slow and bureaucratic and the Kennedy Report itself criticises the existing system. The Government had indicated in *The NHS Plan* that it would look to make changes in the way the NHS handles and responds to clinical negligence claims. Fairness and responsiveness to patients and staff; costs – in excess of £400 million in 1999/2000; and the disincentive to open reporting of error are all areas of concern. For this reason we announced in July 2001 our plans to produce a White Paper early in 2002.

79

The Department of Health's Response to the Report of the Public Inquiry into children's heart surgery at the Bristol Royal Infirmary 1984-1995

5.26 The White Paper will set out reforms to the system for dealing with clinical negligence claims. The Chief Medical Officer is currently leading a committee to look at ways of making the system fairer and faster, not only for patients but also for NHS doctors, nurses and other health care professionals. Views are being sought on possibilities for change to provide the basis for the White Paper, which will give full consideration to a wide range of potential options for reform.

5.27 Whether or not patients wish to pursue complaints or clinical negligence claims, they are entitled to a proper explanation and apology when things go wrong. However, the current system of clinical negligence litigation can act as a barrier to full and frank disclosure. We will be exploring the Kennedy Report's proposal for a duty of candour within the work of the CMO's Committee on Clinical Negligence.

Conclusion

5.28 When things go wrong in health care, they can have devastating consequences: killing and injuring patients, destroying families, undermining the confidence of clinical teams, eroding the reputation of a service and costing large amounts of money. Through the development of a safety culture through clinical governance, the proper training and support of clinicians and through the work of the NPSA, we can act to reduce unnecessary harm, save lives and free up financial and other resources for more and better care to meet the vision of a safe high quality health service which the Kennedy Report and the Government share.

5.29 In responding to the Kennedy Report's recommendations on safety, we will introduce the following changes:

- there will be a single national system of reporting adverse events and 'near misses' through the NPSA;

- from early 2002 the NPSA will analyse the data collected and feed back lessons quickly to the NHS and elsewhere;

- at a local level staff NHS Trusts and PCTs will be encouraged to learn lessons from adverse events rather than seek to allocate blame;

- guidance on root cause analysis will be issued to help NHS Trusts analyse adverse events;

- all staff will be trained to report incidents and to whom;

- work with the Design Council to identify opportunities for design solutions to safety problems;

- we will strengthen accountability arrangements and supervision responsibilities through job plans for consultants to ensure that junior doctors are properly supported and supervised when undertaking new procedures;

- from April 2002 NICE will be responsible for providing the oversight and scrutiny needed for the introduction of new interventional procedures;

- NHS Trusts will receive guidance on the local systems they will need for managing new interventional techniques;

- patients will be told when their treatment is of an experimental nature;

- the use of simulated patients and theatre settings, which allow for development of clinical skills without exposing actual patients to risks, will be expanded; and

- we will introduce a White Paper on the system for dealing with clinical negligence claims early in 2002.

81

The Department of Health's Response to the Report of the Public Inquiry into children's heart surgery at the Bristol Royal Infirmary 1984-1995

Chapter 6

A HEALTH SERVICE WHICH IS WELL LED: MANAGEMENT AND LEADERSHIP

An effective organisation benefits from being clear about how it is led and how this leadership is followed through at every level in the organisation. It is clear about the framework and values within which it operates; about the respective roles, functions and responsibilities of the different players; and it enables the creation of an open and questioning culture which encourages all within it to examine their own practice in the attempt to deliver the highest standards. This chapter sets out our proposals for improving the management and leadership of health bodies at the local level.

6.1   In setting out our agenda for the NHS for the next ten years we have placed at its centre a vision of quality which seeks to address the deep-seated problems of the past, so eloquently described in the Kennedy Report. The ability to deliver safe, effective and high quality care within organisations with the right cultures, the best systems and the most highly skilled and motivated workforce will be the key to meeting this challenge. The health service needs to equip its managers and health professionals with the leadership and management skills essential in developing the new organisational environments which will be needed to achieve a transformation in the quality of patient care. We need to ensure that NHS Trust board and PCT members and the members of the new Strategic Health Authorities are clearer about the role they must play in bringing about the cultural transformation necessary and are themselves well supported and developed for that role.

Developing leadership and management skills

Recommendations 65 - 68, 77

Recommendation 65

An early priority for the new NHS Leadership Centre should be to offer guidelines as to the leadership styles and practices that are acceptable and to be encouraged within the NHS, and those which are not.

Recommendation 66

Steps should be taken to identify and train those within the NHS who have the potential to exercise leadership. There needs to be sustained investment in developing leadership skills at all levels in the NHS.

Recommendation 67

The NHS's investment in developing and funding programmes in leadership skills should be focused on supporting joint education and multi-professional training, open to nurses, doctors, managers and other healthcare professionals.

Recommendation 68

The NHS Leadership Centre should be involved in all stages of the education, training and continuing development of all healthcare professionals.

Recommendation 77

Universities should develop closer links between medical and nursing schools and centres for education and training in health service and public sector management, with a view to enabling all healthcare professionals to learn about management.

6.2   As the Kennedy Report indicates, the approach to developing leadership and management skills, particularly for health professionals, has been patchy in the past. Many health professionals have taken on senior management roles with little training or induction: non-executives have been appointed to NHS Trust boards without a clear understanding of their role; and senior managers have not always had the support and development that they needed to take on the challenge of leading major health care institutions.

6.3   Health organisations need to embrace the concept of leadership. This includes:

* leadership from the top;

83

The Department of Health's Response to the Report of the Public Inquiry into children's heart surgery at the Bristol Royal Infirmary 1984-1995

- empowerment of staff;

- team work;

- prevention, rather than correction of adverse outcomes;

- analysing, simplifying and improving processes;

- commitment to encouraging clinicians into management;

- ensuring greater involvement of women and people from ethnic minority backgrounds in management; and

- a strong patient focus.

This leadership must be provided both by managers at all levels of the organisation, by clinical leaders and by non-executive directors.

6.4　A high quality modern health service needs high quality leaders to provide the vision and values to the organisation; to provide staff with a common and consistent purpose and clear expectations; and to create an environment and ethos which allows the development of an open and honest culture. Without the right leadership we will not make the progress we need to deliver the modern NHS to which we are committed. It is for this reason that we have established the NHS Leadership Centre as part of the NHS Modernisation Agency to develop and support the leaders we need and to build on the leadership capacity we already have. The NHS Leadership Centre will integrate its activities with those of the NHSU.

6.5　Actions already in hand by the NHS Leadership Centre are:

- the development of a values and behaviours framework - local leadership programmes will be designed around it;

- coaching and mentoring for senior staff in the NHS; and

- a new executive director development programme focusing on multi-professional roles and responsibilities. This will bring together medical and nursing directors with colleagues from general management and finance.

6.6   The NHS Leadership Centre will also work with those involved in the education, training and continuing development of health care professionals and with the NHSU to ensure a coherent approach to the development of leadership skills in the NHS.

6.7   Creating truly effective leadership demands a more systematic approach to creating the leaders and managers of the future. We know that education and training programmes are not enough: we know that people need to be given the time to do the job and support to learn and develop the role. Developing leaders means supporting leaders at all levels in the service and across all disciplines. Increasingly many health care professionals will at some time in their career hold formal management roles. Where clinicians take on management roles there needs to be careful consideration of the relationship between clinical and managerial career paths.

6.8   We are working with the NHS Leadership Centre on setting up a national system of succession planning for and development of senior NHS and Department of Health staff. The brief extends to looking at work carried out by other large organisations and identifying best practice.

The role and responsibilities of NHS Trust boards

Recommendations 49 - 56

Recommendation 49

The criteria and process for selection of the executive directors of a trust board must be open and transparent. Appointments should be made on the basis of ability and not on the basis of seniority.

Recommendation 50

The NHS Leadership Centre, in conjunction with trusts, should develop programmes of training and support for clinicians and others who seek to become executive directors.

Recommendation 51

As recommended in *'The NHS Plan'*, there should be an NHS Appointments Commission responsible for the appointment of non-executive directors of NHS trusts, health authorities and primary care trusts.

Recommendation 52

Newly appointed non-executive directors of trusts, health authorities and primary care trusts should receive a programme of induction: this should refer to the principles and values of the NHS and their duties and responsibilities with regard to the quality of care provided by the trust. This programme should be provided through the NHS Leadership Centre.

Recommendation 53

A standard job description should be developed by the NHS for non-executive directors, as proposed in *'The NHS Plan'*.

Recommendation 54

Throughout their period of tenure, non-executive directors should be provided with training, support and advice organised and co-ordinated through the NHS Leadership Centre.

Recommendation 55

The Chairs of trust boards should have a source of independent advice (or mentor) during their period of office, drawn from a pool of experts assembled by the NHS Leadership Centre.

Recommendation 56

Arrangements should be in place in the standing orders of trust boards to provide for proper continuity in the management of the trust's affairs in the period between the cessation of the Chair's term of office and the commencement of that of a successor.

6.9   Strong leadership needs to be a central feature of the NHS and should emanate from the NHS Trust and PCT boards, with an effective mix of executive and non-executive directors whose role is to provide leadership to the organisation, ensure its effective governance and take responsibility for the management and performance of the institution. The BRI Inquiry found this leadership lacking in Bristol and confusion over the role and responsibilities of board members. The Report calls for NHS Trust and PCT boards to lead health care at the local level, with non-executives playing an active role and executive directors appropriately trained for their role. We have already put in hand a number of changes which address this problem.

6.10 The Kennedy Report expresses concern about situations where there is a hiatus between the retirement of a chair and the appointment of a successor. We agree with Professor Kennedy that there should be arrangements in place for the proper and continuing governance of NHS Trusts and PCTs. Model standing orders provide for the deputy chair to take on chairmanship of the board when the chair is not available. The NHS Appointments Commission will ensure that only in rare instances will there be a gap between the retirement of a chair and the appointment of a successor.

6.11 Non-executive directors play a key role in the leadership and management of local health care, and it is right that we should have arrangements in place to recruit and support the best available candidates. The NHS Appointments Commission, which the Kennedy Report endorses, was established on 1 April 2001 under the chairmanship of Sir William Wells with eight Regional Commissioners. It has already made over 600 appointments.

6.12 A standard description of the chair and non-executive role has been developed and is now used in the recruitment of all chairs and non-executives. An induction guide for chairs and non-executive directors is being developed by the NHS Leadership Centre and the NHS Appointments Commission. It will be published in January 2002. The NHS Leadership Centre has gathered a considerable amount of information and knowledge on people with the skills and expertise to mentor others and, together with the Appointments Commission, will act as broker to bring suitable individuals together. The National Clinical Governance Support Team is running a programme specifically aimed at the strategic leadership of clinical governance by NHS Trust boards.

6.13 *Appointments to the Most Senior Posts in the NHS* (EL(97)84), issued in December 1997, sets out arrangements to ensure that the appointment of executive directors is rigorous. But we also recognise that there is a need for effective training and support for those already in senior posts. The NHS Leadership Centre is introducing an executive director development programme in January 2002 and will support the development programme at local level.

87

The Department of Health's Response to the Report of the Public Inquiry into children's heart surgery at the Bristol Royal Infirmary 1984-1995

The management of the NHS at local level

Recommendations 43, 48

Recommendation 43

The contractual relationship between trusts and consultants should be redefined. The trust must provide the consultant with the time, space and the necessary tools to do the job. Consultants must accept that the time spent in the hospital and what they do in that time must be explicitly set out.

Recommendation 48

The security of tenure of the chief executive and senior managers of trusts should be on a par with that of other senior professionals in the NHS.

6.14 The Kennedy Report calls for a clearer contractual relationship between NHS Trusts and consultants in which the expected commitment and behaviours are clearly set out in return for the support and resources required to do the job. We recognise and support the view that the relationship and expectations placed on NHS staff by their employing NHS Trust should be made more explicit. We are in the process of making clearer this relationship across a number of staff groups and new contracts are currently being negotiated for consultants and GPs.

6.15 Our proposals for the new consultant contract will ensure that job planning provides the basis for a stronger, unambiguous framework of contractual obligations. Job plans cover all aspects of a consultant's practice in the NHS and will set out clearly the consultant's time and service commitments. Employers will be expected to ensure that consultants have the facilities and other support needed to carry out the responsibilities and duties set out in the job plans.

6.16 Professor Kennedy recognises the central role managers play in the delivery of the NHS and recommends that they should be treated as health care professionals, deserving of the same respect and carrying the same responsibility for ensuring their competence as the other health professionals employed in the NHS. We think there is a strong case for modernising and streamlining contractual arrangements for senior managers and plan to consult on a new framework for delivering this in the near future. This will include proposals to ensure that all senior managerial contracts are without term and set out the circumstances in which a contract may be brought to an end.

Clinicians who hold managerial positions

Recommendations 92 - 98

Recommendation 92

Where clinicians hold managerial roles which extend beyond their immediate clinical practice, sufficient protected time in the form of allocated sessions must be made available for them to carry out that managerial role.

Recommendation 93

Any clinician, before appointment to a managerial role, must demonstrate the managerial competence to undertake what is required in that role: training and support should be made available by trusts and primary care trusts.

Recommendation 94

Clinicians should not be required or expected to hold managerial roles on bases other than competence for the job. For example, seniority or being next in turn are not appropriate criteria for the appointment of clinicians to managerial roles.

Recommendation 95

The professional and financial incentives for senior clinicians to undertake full-time senior managerial roles should be reviewed: the aim should be to enable senior clinicians to move into a full-time managerial role, and subsequently, if they so wish, to move back into clinical practice after appropriate retraining and revalidation.

Recommendation 96

To protect patients, in the case of clinicians who take on managerial roles but wish to continue to practise as clinicians, experts together with managers from the NHS should issue advice as to the minimum level of regular clinical practice necessary to enable a clinician to provide care of a good quality. Clinicians not maintaining this level of practice should not be entitled to offer clinical care. This rule should also apply to all other clinicians who, for whatever reason, are not in full-time practice, and not only to those in part-time managerial roles.

Recommendation 97

To facilitate the movement of clinicians in and out of managerial positions, the proposed systems for the revalidation (and re-registration) of doctors, nurses and professions allied to medicine should distinguish between professionals who are managers and also maintaining a clinical practice and those who are not. Those who are not maintaining a clinical practice should be entitled to obtain the appropriate revalidation (and re-registration) to restart a clinical practice, after retraining, and should be assisted in doing so.

> **Recommendation 98**
>
> **The relevant professional regulatory bodies should make rules varying the professional duties of those professionals, whose registration they hold, who are in full-time managerial roles, so as to take account of the fact that, while occupying such roles, they do not undertake responsibility for the care of patients.**

6.17 The Kennedy Report recognises the importance of clinicians' involvement in managerial roles and calls for such appointments to be based on appointment criteria and adequately supported. We believe that in a modern health service clinicians should continue to play a strong role in its management and in so doing ensure that clinical needs are properly taken into account in decision making.

6.18 The proposals for job planning in the new consultant contract will ensure that management responsibilities are considered alongside clinical duties and reflected in timetabled job plans.

6.19 Clinical director and medical director development programmes are to be rolled out this year by the NHS Leadership Centre with a strong emphasis on the skills required to lead and manage change with colleagues. The newly introduced consultant appraisal process will provide evidence for identifying an individual's potential for these roles and personal development plans will highlight development actions. We plan to use the values and behaviours framework for leadership when selecting leaders of the future and clinical managers will be selected on the basis of skills and potential, not on the basis of seniority.

6.20 We agree with the recommendations of the Kennedy Report that systems should be designed to encourage clinicians to move between clinical and management roles and back again. We already have in place systems to take account of the financial and professional issues involved. Appraisal and better systems for professional development and career planning mean that clinicians will be better supported in management roles and that revalidation and re-registration will be more straightforward. Thus movement between clinical practice and management will be encouraged and supported.

6.21 We have given careful thought to the Kennedy recommendations dealing with minimum levels of regular clinical practice and an alternative form of registration for health care professionals in management roles. We strongly endorse the view that all professionals have a duty to act within their competence. This is enshrined in the professional codes and registration; in clinical governance; and in the systems for appraisal and revalidation and re-registration. There are, however, an enormous number of specialties and variation in practice and we do not believe it would be possible as Professor Kennedy suggests to prescribe a pattern which would suit every case. Rather it is for the individual to ensure that they are competent to practise in their chosen field. This will be tested regularly through clinical governance procedures, annual appraisal and through providing sufficient evidence as part of revalidation or re-registration.

6.22 We recognise that there are particular difficulties facing doctors outside substantive employment (for example part-time doctors and locums) and as part of the introduction of appraisal for NHS doctors we are setting up advisory and support structures which will help them address any concerns about the appropriateness of their practice.

6.23 Most health professionals, even when they are in full-time management, need to retain their professional status and wish to work according to their professional ethos. We do not therefore propose to follow the route of alternative forms of registration which the Kennedy Report recommends.

Conclusion

6.24 We are clear that strong leadership and good governance are central to driving the cultural changes set out in the Kennedy Report and our vision for the NHS. We have started a programme to support the leadership skills that are already in place, to extend them and to embed them more deeply throughout the service.

6.25 In responding to the Kennedy Report's recommendations on management and leadership, we will:

- establish the NHSU from 2003;

- ensure the NHS Leadership Centre/ NHS Modernisation Agency and NHSU work to support and develop leaders throughout the NHS;

- ensure all non-executive and chair appointments to NHS Trust and PCT boards are made by the NHS Appointments Commission;

- introduce an executive director development programme in January 2002;

- commence clinical director and medical director development programmes from January 2002 to support clinicians in management;

- produce an induction guide for non-executive directors in 2002;

- ensure mentors are available for NHS Trust and PCT chairs;

- ensure contract changes make more explicit the expectations placed on NHS staff by their employing NHS Trusts and PCTs; and

- enable professionals regularly to reassess their competence both clinically and for any management duties though consultant appraisal, revalidation and re-registration.

THE REGULATION AND EDUCATION OF HEALTH CARE PROFESSIONALS

This chapter considers the means by which well-trained and competent health care staff are developed to meet the needs of patients in a modern NHS and the system of regulation for enforcing those standards.

7.1 The quality of care delivered to patients depends crucially on the calibre of staff working in the NHS. This means identifying the needs of the service now and for the future, setting clear standards, and working with the training organisations to ensure education and training programmes meet those standards. NHS patients need to know that the staff that care for them are well-trained and competent; education, training and development must meet the needs of the NHS now and in the future; and above all it must produce and support health care professionals who are equipped with skills, knowledge and values set out in both *The NHS Plan* and the Kennedy Report.

Our approach to regulation

Recommendations 41, 69 - 74, 90

Recommendation 41
The various bodies whose purpose it is to assure the quality of care in the NHS (for example, CHI and NICE) and the competence of healthcare professionals (for example, the GMC and the Nursing and Midwifery Council) must themselves be independent of and at arm's-length from the DoH.

Recommendations 69
Regulation of healthcare professionals is not just about disciplinary matters. It should be understood as encapsulating all of the systems which combine to assure the competence of healthcare professionals: education, registration, training, CPD and revalidation as well as disciplinary matters.

The Department of Health's Response to the Report of the Public Inquiry into children's heart surgery at the Bristol Royal Infirmary 1984-1995

Recommendation 70

For *each* group of healthcare professionals (doctors, nurses and midwives, the professions allied to medicine, and managers) there should be one body charged with overseeing *all* aspects relating to the regulation of professional life: education, registration, training, CPD, revalidation and discipline. The bodies should be: for doctors, the GMC; for nurses and midwives, the new Nursing and Midwifery Council; for the professions allied to medicine, the re-formed professional body for those professions; and for senior healthcare managers, a new professional body.

Recommendation 71

In addition, a single body should be charged with the overall co-ordination of the various professional bodies and with integrating the various systems of regulation. It should be called the Council for the Regulation of Healthcare Professionals. (In effect, this is the body currently proposed in *'The NHS Plan'*, and referred to as the Council of Healthcare Regulators.)

Recommendation 72

The Council for the Regulation of Healthcare Professionals should be established as a matter of priority. It should have a statutory basis. It should report to Parliament. It should have a broadly-based membership, consisting of representatives of the bodies which regulate the various groups of healthcare professionals, of the NHS, and of the general public.

Recommendation 73

The Council for the Regulation of Healthcare Professionals should have formal powers to require bodies which regulate the separate groups of healthcare professionals to conform to principles of good regulation. It should act as a source of guidance and of good practice. It should seek to ensure that in practice the bodies which regulate healthcare professionals behave in a consistent and broadly similar manner.

Recommendation 74

It should be a priority for the Council for the Regulation of Healthcare Professionals to promote common curricula and shared learning across the professions.

Recommendation 90

The new Council for the Regulation of Healthcare Professionals should take as a further priority an early review of the various systems of revalidation and re-registration to ensure that they are sufficiently rigorous, and in alignment both with each other and with other initiatives to protect the public. The Council should also seek ways to incorporate managers (as healthcare professionals) into the systems of CPD, appraisal and revalidation.

7.2   The public and patients are entitled to expect that the health care professionals with whom they come in contact are well-regulated and that there is consistency across the professional boundaries. The Kennedy Report calls for a single body for each health care profession, charged with overseeing all aspects of the regulation of professional life and a single body to co-ordinate the various professional bodies. We signalled our intention to modernise the regulation of health care professions in *The NHS Plan* in July 2000. In August 2001 we published a consultation document *Modernising Regulation in the Health Professions*, outlining our proposals for the creation of the Council for the Regulation of Health Care Professionals. The new Council will work with the regulatory bodies to build and manage a strong system of self-regulation which:

- explicitly puts patients first;

- is open and transparent and allows for robust public scrutiny;

- ensures that existing regulatory bodies act in a more consistent manner;

- provides for greater integration and co-ordination between the regulatory bodies and the sharing of good practice and information;

- adheres to the principles of good regulation set out in *Supporting Doctors, Protecting Patients* published by the Department of Health in 1999; and

- promotes continuous improvements through the setting of new performance targets and monitoring.

7.3   These proposals are designed to replace the current fragmented arrangements for the regulation of health professions with a modern framework that puts patients at the heart of the process; gives them stronger safeguards and protection against poor performance; and rebuilds public confidence in the ability of the regulatory bodies to set acceptable standards for the quality of health professionals' work and to deal effectively and fairly with individuals who do not meet these standards.

95

The Department of Health's Response to the Report of the Public Inquiry into children's heart surgery at the Bristol Royal Infirmary 1984-1995

Accountability and membership

7.4   It is essential that the health care regulatory bodies work together to develop common approaches across the professions and agree standards that put patients' interests clearly at the centre of all they do. The regulatory bodies need to reflect the changing nature and character of the NHS workforce and the way that health care is delivered on the ground. This can be best achieved under the effective co-ordination of the new Council, with the support of reformed regulatory bodies.

7.5   We are working with the existing bodies to ensure that they become more responsive to the views of stakeholders so that they meet reasonable patient expectations and the changes in service delivery that have taken place in recent years. We have consulted widely on the reform of the regulation of nursing, midwifery and health visiting and the allied health professions. Parliament has recently confirmed our proposals for the establishment of the Nursing and Midwifery Council and the Health Professions Council. We are discussing proposals with the General Medical Council (GMC) for the reform of its governance and changes to the registration of doctors including the introduction of revalidation and fitness to practise. We will be reforming the General Dental Council, introducing a compulsory continuous professional development for dentists and reforming disciplinary procedures for pharmacists. The proposals add up to the biggest reform of health care professional self-regulation and demonstrate our commitment to providing an independent statutory framework for health care professions in which the public and patients can have full confidence.

7.6   We have given careful thought to the view that the various bodies whose purpose is to assure the competence of health care professionals should be independent of and at arm's length from the Department of Health. Regulation of professional staff goes beyond employment in the NHS and regulates the competence and ability of an individual to work in a range of settings both in NHS and private practice. We accept that regulation of professionals should properly be at arm's length from Ministers. We propose that the Council for the Regulation of Health Care Professionals should be accountable to Parliament. The regulatory bodies will be accountable to the new Council and through it to Parliament. Arrangements for each body will be reviewed once the new Council is in place.

Managers

> **Recommendation 91**
>
> **Managers as healthcare professionals should be subject to the same obligations as other healthcare professionals, including being subject to a regulatory body and professional code of practice.**

7.7 Careful consideration has been given to the recommendation in the Kennedy Report that managers should themselves be subject to a new regulatory professional body. We endorse the view that managers should be subject to a code of behaviour and have the appropriate skills and competence to discharge their roles. Since the events at Bristol, managers have become subject to a wide range of monitoring and inspection systems. CHI explicitly inspects the statutory duty of quality placed on chief executives through its clinical governance reviews and service managers are now explicitly accountable for the quality of patient care and patient services.

7.8 We agree, that more needs to be done to improve the quality of NHS management. Raising standards and raising the value of managers go hand in hand and will lead to the better management of services for the benefit of patients. We do not think it practicable, however, at this stage to establish a formal regulatory body. Rather we propose to establish the safeguards for patients and the service through the introduction of a seven point action plan, which will include:

- a new core contract for NHS senior managers;

- a new mandatory code of conduct, incorporated into the employment contract, setting out the duties and style of management and leadership appropriate in the modern NHS;

- a new statement of the skills, knowledge and behaviour expected of NHS managers, against which they will be explicitly assessed;

- the introduction of formal Continuing Professional Development (CPD) incorporated into the new contract of employment;

- strengthening the selection process for appointments to the most senior management posts;

- a new succession planning system; and

97

The Department of Health's Response to the Report of the Public Inquiry into children's heart surgery at the Bristol Royal Infirmary 1984-1995

•   exploring the feasibility of an accreditation scheme for NHS managers.

The education of health care professionals

Recommendations 75, 76, 78 - 80

Recommendation 75

Pilot schemes should be established to develop and evaluate the feasibility of making the first year's course of undergraduate education common to all those wishing to become healthcare professionals.

Recommendation 76

Universities should develop closer links between medical schools and schools of nursing education with a view to providing more joint education between medical and nursing students.

Recommendation 78

Access to medical schools should be widened to include people from diverse academic and socio-economic backgrounds. Those with qualifications in other areas of healthcare and those with an educational background in subjects other than science, who have the ability and wish to do so, should have greater opportunities than is presently the case, to enter medical schools.

Recommendation 79

The attributes of a good doctor, as set down in the GMC's *'Good Medical Practice'*, must inform every aspect of the selection criteria and curricula of medical schools.

Recommendation 80

The NHS and the public should be involved in (a) establishing the criteria for selection and (b) the selection of those to be educated as doctors, nurses and as other healthcare professionals.

7.9   The Kennedy Report calls for a broadening of the social and academic base from which health care professionals are drawn and for more joint training courses between professions to foster multi-disciplinary working. We are committed to widening access to medical schools. Our programme to increase the number of places by 2010 is based on medical schools demonstrating an active commitment to recruiting students from a broad range of social and ethnic backgrounds, to reflect the patterns of the population that they serve. The increases included a number of places for existing graduates to enter shorter courses, as part of our strategy to encourage people from a broader range of backgrounds, including other health care professionals, to move into medicine. We are exploring other means of attracting people from backgrounds which have not traditionally gone into medicine.

7.10 We recognise that there should be greater public involvement as recommended in the Kennedy Report in the selection of those entering training as health care professionals. NHS managers and practitioners are already frequently involved in aspects of the selection process for nursing, midwifery and allied health professional students. We are taking steps to strengthen this further through Workforce Development Confederations and following the strategies for nursing, midwifery and health visiting *(Making a Difference),* allied health professionals *(Meeting the Challenge)* and health care scientists *(Making the Change).* Whilst it is for the regulatory bodies and higher education institutions to set their requirements for admission to professional training, we are committed to encouraging broad and diverse participation in selection procedures.

7.11 The aim of undergraduate medical education is to produce doctors who are able to meet the nation's present and future health care needs. The expansion of places in existing universities, together with the brand new medical schools will create generations of new doctors equipped to meet the challenges of twenty first century medicine. New, modern curricula will mean that tomorrow's doctors will be skilled not just in management and treatment of disease, but in communicating with their patients, in assuring the quality of the care they provide, in realising the potential of e-medicine and in helping people stay healthy. No longer will medical education be a 'doctor only world', students of medicine, nursing and other professions will have more systematic opportunities to learn together in practice based settings, supporting better teamwork, which will be essential in the day to day care of patients.

7.12 We need to make full use of new developments in teaching methods. As part of their CPD, doctors are increasingly using the Internet to learn about clinical advances in other countries and to communicate rapidly with professional colleagues. Other electronic advances in methods of training doctors include an electronic arm on which doctors can practise taking blood and a computer generated surgical theatre to accustom doctors to theatre practices, which, for example, allows them to learn and experiment with different stitching techniques without risk to an actual patient.

Common learning for health care professionals

Recommendations 19, 57 - 64

Recommendation 19

Healthcare professionals responsible for the care of any particular patient must communicate effectively with each other. The aim must be to avoid giving the patient conflicting advice and information.

Recommendation 57

Greater priority than at present should be given to non-clinical aspects of care in six key areas in the education, training and continuing professional development of healthcare professionals:

- skills in communicating with patients and with colleagues;
- education about the principles and organisation of the NHS, and about how care is managed, and the skills required for management;
- the development of teamwork;
- shared learning across professional boundaries;
- clinical audit and reflective practice; and
- leadership.

Recommendation 58

Competence in non-clinical aspects of caring for patients should be formally assessed as part of the process of obtaining an initial professional qualification, whether as a doctor, a nurse or some other healthcare professional.

Recommendation 59

Education in communication skills must be an essential part of the education of all healthcare professionals. Communication skills include the ability to engage with patients on an emotional level, to listen, to assess how much information a patient wants to know, and to convey information with clarity and sympathy.

Recommendations 60

Communication skills must also include the ability to engage with and respect the views of fellow healthcare professionals.

Recommendation 61

The education, training and Continuing Professional Development (CPD) of all healthcare professionals should include joint courses between the professions.

> **Recommendation 62**
>
> **There should be more opportunities than at present for multi-professional teams to learn, train and develop together.**
>
> **Recommendation 63**
>
> **All those preparing for a career in clinical care should receive some education in the management of healthcare, the health service and the skills required for management.**
>
> **Recommendation 64**
>
> **Greater opportunities should be created for managers and clinicians to 'shadow' one another for short periods to learn about their respective roles and work pressures.**

7.13 We fully support the Kennedy view that health care professionals need to be aware of and respect each others' roles if they are to deliver modern health care together. *The NHS Plan* has already signalled our commitment in this area and we have already invited proposals from 'leading edge' Higher Education Institutions/Workforce Development Confederation partnership sites to develop more undergraduate health care professionals programmes which incorporate more common and shared learning elements throughout the curriculum. This is key to our commitment to have common learning programmes in place for all health professions by 2004. It will also help to develop closer links between medical, nursing and other health professional programmes in university departments.

7.14 Central to this is the development of communication skills, not only between the health care professionals and patients but also between professionals themselves, both within and outwith the NHS, as part of multi-disciplinary working. Only by engaging with and respecting the views of others can a true partnership be entered into and high quality care be delivered. We recognise that all professionals need an understanding of the contribution they each make to providing a safe, high quality health service. Clinicians can no longer ignore the wider resourcing and management framework within which they operate: managers must also have a proper understanding of what is needed to deliver a clinical service which meets patients' needs and expectations.

7.15 To underpin recent decisions on major increases in medical school places, all universities were required to describe how their proposals would underpin the development of multi-professional education - to ensure that care would be delivered to patients by the staff best able to give it by skill rather than professional label and to ensure that the doctors of the future are team workers.

7.16 We accept, therefore, the Kennedy recommendations that greater priority should be given to non-clinical aspects of care in the education, training and development of those working within the NHS. As part of *The NHS Plan* action agenda we are working with the regulatory and professional bodies and the educational providers to ensure that these skills, knowledge and values are included in all NHS funded professional programmes, and undergraduate medical, nursing, dental and pharmacy training by the end of 2002.

Post-qualification training and continuing professional development

Recommendations 81 - 84

Recommendation 81

In relation to doctors, we endorse the proposal to establish a Medical Education Standards Board (MESB), to co-ordinate postgraduate medical training. The MESB should be part of and answerable to the GMC which should have a wider role.

Recommendation 82

CPD, being fundamental to the quality of care provided to patients, should be compulsory for all healthcare professionals.

Recommendation 83

Trusts and primary care trusts should provide incentives to encourage healthcare professionals to maintain and develop their skills. The contract (or, in the case of GPs, other relevant mechanism) between the trust and the healthcare professional should provide for the funding of CPD and should stipulate the time which the trust will make available for CPD.

Recommendation 84

Trusts and primary care trusts must take overall responsibility through an agreed plan for their employees' use of the time allocated to CPD. They must seek to ensure that the resources deployed for CPD contribute towards meeting the needs of the trust and of its patients, as well as meeting the professional aspirations of individual healthcare professionals.

7.17 The delivery of modern health care is highly skilled and complex: the limits of what can be achieved in modern medicine and health care are continuously expanding and the demands placed on health care professionals are increasingly more challenging. In this context, the importance of continuing development and life long learning for all who work in the NHS is self evident.

7.18 The Kennedy Report recommends making the proposed Medical Education Standards Board (MESB) part of and answerable to the GMC. After careful thought we have decided not to accept this recommendation. The use of the considerable resources which go into post-graduate medical education should reflect the needs of the service, as well as individual clinicians and it is right that there should be closer ties between the MESB and the NHS as the Kennedy Report suggests.

7.19 The MESB will set standards for post-graduate medical education and training. To become a consultant or a general practitioner, doctors will have to be assessed by the Board to see whether they have met those standards. For the first time, the Board will bring together patients, the NHS and the medical profession in making key decisions about how doctors are trained. The Board will provide a managed and quality assured framework for the training of doctors, to ensure that doctors get the training they need to deliver the services patients deserve. Our detailed proposals for the Board are being published separately.

7.20 CPD is clearly an important component in maintaining and updating skills and expertise. The Kennedy Report recommends that it should be compulsory. All regulated professionals have a duty to maintain their knowledge and keep their skills up to date as part of the requirement of their professional code and failure to do so puts their continued registration (and hence employment) at risk. We believe that CPD requirements should be identified on the basis of the needs of individuals, within the context of the needs of the organisation and local clinical guidance. The key focus for this is the formal appraisal process together with a personal development plan agreed between the individual professional and their manager with the commitment of the necessary time and resources. Our proposals for modernising the NHS pay system require that appraisal and development should become a regular part of working life for all NHS staff, and the pay modernisation proposals in *Agenda for Change* suggest a link between appraisal and pay progression to reward staff who develop new skills and knowledge.

7.21 In April 2001, as part of our commitment to CPD in *The NHS Plan* we allocated £20m to support development of the learning infrastructure for CPD. The NHS Lifelong Learning Framework and the implementation of the NHS Improving Working Lives Standard will further reinforce our plans in this area. Workforce Development Confederations will lead this work locally, ensuring that national criteria for investment fit with local needs and priorities and cover all settings including primary care. The National Clinical Governance Support Team launched a programme in October 2001 which will support staff in developing communication and team working skills and shared learning across professional boundaries.

Appraisal

Recommendations 85 - 87

Recommendation 85

Periodic appraisal should be compulsory for all healthcare professionals. The requirement to participate in appraisal should be included in the contract of employment.

Recommendation 86

The commitment in *'The NHS Plan'* to introduce regular appraisal for hospital consultants must be implemented as soon as possible.

Recommendation 87

The requirement to undergo periodic appraisal should also be incorporated into GPs' terms of service.

7.22 The Kennedy Report rightly highlights the importance of appraisal. Appraisal is an essential tool in reviewing performance and is a crucial component of reflective practice and the systems which assure competence, quality and the safety of care. Appraisal for consultants was introduced on 1 April 2001 and GP appraisal is under negotiation. Appraisal for all other NHS doctors will be rolled out in the coming year. All staff should already have a personal development plan and we are committed to introducing an appraisal process which will cover all NHS staff. Development work is now beginning and we intend to build on existing good practice.

Revalidation

Recommendations 88, 89

Recommendation 88

Periodic revalidation, whereby healthcare professionals demonstrate that they remain fit to practise in their chosen profession, should be compulsory for all healthcare professionals. The requirement to participate in periodic revalidation should be included in the contract of employment.

Recommendation 89

The public, as well as the employer and the relevant professional group, must be involved in the processes of revalidation.

7.23 The Kennedy Report calls for compulsory rigorous systems of revalidation and registration, with public involvement in the process of revalidation. We are already committed to the principle of revalidation and are actively working with the GMC to introduce revalidation for all doctors. Medical revalidation includes lay involvement in assessing individual doctors and this should be a benchmark for other professions. The Council for the Regulation of Health Care Professionals will have a role in the development of common approaches to revalidation across the professions.

Clinical excellence awards

Recommendation 44

The system of Distinction Awards for hospital consultants should be examined to determine whether it could be used to provide greater incentives than exist at present for providing good quality of care to patients. The possibility of its extension to include junior hospital doctors should be explored.

7.24 The Kennedy Report draws attention to the role of clinical excellence awards in motivating doctors. We issued proposals for consultation last year on a new NHS Clinical Excellence Award Scheme to replace the current distinction awards and discretionary points schemes. We will be implementing a new scheme designed to reward those who make the biggest contribution to delivering and improving local health services. The new scheme will provide a further powerful incentive to high quality practice by using assessment criteria based on patient centred service and care. Patients will be represented on local awards

105

The Department of Health's Response to the Report of the Public Inquiry into children's heart surgery at the Bristol Royal Infirmary 1984-1995

committees. Fuller proposals are being developed in the light of consultation and the Kennedy recommendations will be taken into account as part of this work.

Professional codes of conduct

> ### Recommendations 45, 46
>
> #### Recommendation 45
> The doctors' Code of Professional Practice, as set down in the GMC's *'Good Medical Practice'*, should be incorporated into the contract of employment between doctors and trusts. In the case of GPs, the terms of service should be amended to incorporate the Code.
>
> #### Recommendation 46
> The relevant codes of practice for nurses, for professions allied to medicine and for managers should be incorporated into their contracts of employment with hospital trusts or primary care trusts.

7.25 The Kennedy Report recommends that the codes of professional conduct should be included in the contracts of employment for health professionals, with employers dealing with breaches independently of the actions of the professional body. The required national documentation for consultants' contracts explicitly included the headings in *Good Medical Practice*, so that evidence against all these areas can be considered during appraisal and then by the GMC during its own revalidation process, due to start in 2003/4. The same principles will apply to other NHS doctors.

7.26 Other health professionals have contracts of employment based on the premise that they are properly registered with their regulatory body which itself requires them to meet their professional code of practice, and a professional code of practice for managers is being developed. Compliance with professional codes of conduct are therefore already implicit in employment contracts: we do not believe that we need to go further.

Discipline

> ### Recommendations 47, 104
>
> #### Recommendation 47
> **Trusts should be able to deal as employers with breaches of the relevant professional code by a healthcare professional, independently of any action which the relevant professional body may take.**
>
> #### Recommendation 104
> **In the exercise of their disciplinary function the professional regulatory bodies must adopt a more flexible approach towards what constitutes misconduct. They must deal with cases, as far as possible, at a local level and must have available a range of actions which both serve the interests of the public and the needs of the professional.**

7.27 The regulation and disciplining of health care professionals is a shared responsibility between the employer and the regulatory bodies. We support the view that local employers should be able to deal with breaches of the relevant professional code by a health care professional. New guidance is being prepared to ensure that employers take into account professional codes of practice in their local codes of conduct.

7.28 *Supporting doctors, protecting patients*, recognises that early intervention by health authorities, NHS Trusts and PCTs is needed when concerns about a doctor's practice first arise and before patients are harmed. The National Clinical Assessment Authority (NCAA) will assist health authorities, NHS Trusts and PCTs achieve this. We intend that its scope will be extended to include dentistry and we will also give consideration to extending this approach, under similar arrangements, to other health care professions. Our proposals for the new Nursing and Midwifery and Health Professions Councils include the expectation that they will both develop and operate their policies in partnership with employers.

7.29 In cases where local action has not been able to ensure the protection of the public the matter must be reported to the appropriate regulatory body. We envisage a key role for the Council for the Regulation of Health Care Professionals in ensuring that efficient and effective mechanisms are in place for protecting the public from unacceptable risks presented by those health professionals who are, for whatever reason, unfit to practise.

107

The Department of Health's Response to the Report of the Public Inquiry into children's heart surgery at the Bristol Royal Infirmary 1984-1995

Conclusion

7.30 It is essential that the public should have confidence in the system of professional self-regulation and the competence of the health care professionals involved in their care. We agree that the process of regulation should be at arm's length from government and that there should be greater public involvement in the regulatory processes. But assuring competence is a continuous activity, and one which has a strong relationship with the quality of service we wish the NHS to deliver. For this reason we are committed to continuing professional development and lifelong learning for all staff, linked to systematic appraisals, personal development plans and revalidation. In this way the public can be confident that the individual is appropriately registered with his or her professional body, that skills have been updated to take account of changing clinical practice and that this is a continuing and ongoing process which recognises changes and development in clinical practice over time.

7.31 In responding to the Kennedy report's recommendations we will: -

- establish in the NHS Reform and Health Care Professions Bill a new Council for the Regulation of Health Care Professionals to strengthen and co-ordinate the system of professional self-regulation;

- reform the current arrangements for the regulation of individual health care professions so that patients will be at the heart of professional regulation;

- consult on a new core contract for NHS senior managers, and a mandatory code of conduct;

- widen access to medical schools and increase the number of places by 1,000 by the end of 2002;

- ensure greater public involvement in the selection of those entering training as health care professionals;

- make changes in the education of medical students to produce doctors equipped to meet the challenges of twenty first century medicine;

- ensure a core curriculum on communication, NHS principles and organisation is introduced by the end of 2002;

- develop and evaluate common learning programmes across all Higher Education Institutions by 2004;

- give greater priority to non-clinical aspects of care in the education, training and continuing development of those working in the NHS;

- establish the Medical Education and Standards Board to set standards for post-graduate medical education and training;

- identify CPD requirements on the basis of individual need to ensure staff maintain their skills and knowledge. The LifeLong Learning Framework was published in November 2001;

- spend £20m on CPD this year with more planned for the future through the NHS Lifelong Learning Framework and the NHS Improved Working Lives Standard;

- ensure appraisal for all doctors is introduced by the end of 2002;

- support revalidation by the GMC for all doctors and encourage its extension to all health care professionals;

- implement the NHS Clinical Excellence Awards Scheme in 2003 which will provide greater incentives for high quality, patient centred practice;

- issue new guidance on disciplinary procedures to support local employers in dealing with breaches of the relevant professional code by a health care professional; and

- support the NCAA to assist NHS Trusts and PCTs when concerns about a doctor's practice first arise and before patients are harmed.

Chapter 8

INFORMATION FOR DECISION MAKING AND THE MONITORING OF PERFORMANCE

Any complex organisation needs to be clear about its purpose and objectives and needs information to tell it how far it is meeting those objectives. The NHS is a highly complex organisation. It needs information to enable patients to make informed decisions about their own care; to inform clinicians' judgements to enable them to deliver the best care possible; and to allow the assessment of services against agreed standards to ensure that the NHS continues to treat over a million people each day in a way which is safe, using the resources available - whether staff, facilities or finance - in the most effective ways possible.

8.1   The Kennedy Report is very clear about the importance of high quality, timely information. It recognises that the exchange and provision of information is at the core of an open and honest relationship between health care professionals and patients; that information about performance in the NHS is the basic building block of any system of standards and quality; that information needs to be analysed and used to inform practice; and that to deliver this the NHS needs the right skills and IT infrastructure.

8.2   The NHS needs good information on the nature, quality and performance of its services for a range of important purposes:

 •   to enable patients to make informed choices about the services they wish to use and about their own treatment;

 •   to allow health professionals and patients to review options and design a plan of care;

 •   to allow the performance of services to be assessed against agreed goals and targets, to make comparisons between different local services, and to benchmark against exemplar services and best practice;

- to assure the quality of services and seek opportunities for improvements in the quality of care;

- to identify unsafe practices and situations so that risk for patients can be reduced;

- to underpin appraisal, assessment and revalidation of individual professionals;

- to allow public reporting of health service performance to fulfil a duty of accountability to the taxpayer;

- to evaluate models of care and to promote innovation; and

- to assess the health status of the population and identify scope for the promotion of health and prevention of disease.

8.3 Information must be:

- valid - measures what it seeks to measure;

- relevant - measures what is important;

- accurate - robust against criticisms of unreliability;

- up to date - gives accurate, timely information to allow appropriate interventions;

- easily accessible - is readily available in a convenient form to those who wish to access it; and

- well presented - can be readily understood by those who need to use it.

8.4 If the NHS is to be truly patient centred and patients are to be involved wherever possible in decisions about their treatment and care then patients should be offered full, accurate, understandable, timely information about their condition, its prognosis, the treatment options and the associated risks and benefits.

8.5 Patients should also be offered understandable, timely, accurate, relevant information about the quality of care available to them in a particular NHS organisation, and how it compares with standards of good quality and performance elsewhere. This should include information about the outcomes of care as well as information about other relevant aspects of quality such as patients' experience. And wherever possible patients and their families should have a chance to take information away with them, to reflect upon information and to ask questions. Good quality information also forms the basis for patients to make informed choices about their care.

8.6   At the moment people do not always get the information they need. There are a number of reasons for this including:

- the information does not exist – for example relevant data about quality of care may not have been collected;

- the information exists but is not known or accessible to clinician or patient – for example a clinician may not know about an important advance in clinical science, or may not have access to the results of relevant tests performed elsewhere;

- the information is known by clinicians but they may lack the inclination, skill or time to communicate it clearly to the patient or the patient may not understand the risks as explained;

- there may be specific barriers to communication – e.g. an English speaking clinician and a non-English speaking patient; and

- what clinicians think they have said may not always be what patients think they have heard. And, similarly, information provided verbally may be forgotten.

8.7   All of these issues must be tackled. As yet neither the NHS nor any other health care system in the world has done so successfully. But it is our intention that the NHS should be the first national health care system to do so routinely, systematically and comprehensively. This is a major challenge – but a challenge that will transform the NHS for the better.

8.8   If the care we offer to patients is to be of the highest quality we need to know the outcomes associated with different procedures. To do this we must have in place an effective system of monitoring clinical care through audit at a local level, and the ability to undertake national surveillance to identify both where there may be problems and where there is excellence.

Investing in information

Recommendations 148, 149, 154

Recommendation 148

The current 'dual' system of collecting data in the NHS in separate administrative and multiple clinical systems is wasteful and anachronistic. A single approach to collecting data should be adopted, which clinicians can trust and use and from which information about both clinical and administrative performance can be derived.

Recommendation 149

Steps should be taken nationally and locally to build the confidence of clinicians in the data recorded in the Patient Administration Systems in trusts (which is subsequently aggregated nationally to form the Hospital Episode Statistics). Such steps should include the establishment by trusts of closer working arrangements between clinicians and clinical coding staff.

Recommendation 154

The need to invest in world-class IT systems must be recognised so that the fundamental principles of data collection, validation and management can be observed: that data be collected only once; that the data be part and parcel of systems used to support healthcare professionals in their care of patients; and that trusts and the teams of healthcare professionals receive feedback when data on their services are aggregated.

8.9 Patients, clinicians, managers, analysts and researchers all need good quality information and ready access to modern information and communication technology if the NHS is to reform the services it provides and improve the quality of care. Information and IT underpins delivery of *The NHS Plan*.

8.10 *Information for Health* (published in September 1998) and updated in *Building the Information Core: Implementing the NHS Plan* (January 2001) describes the programme for transforming the handling of information in the NHS. But investment in delivering improved information is a long-term strategy and will take some years to provide the information needed by patients, clinicians and managers.

8.11 A central feature of *Information for Health* is the development of electronic patient records. By 2005 these will provide the basis for a single approach to collecting data for clinical and administrative purposes and for performance assessment. But of equal value is the cultural change their introduction will foster: for the first time patients will have routine access to their records in a way which will support the development of a more open and honest relationship with the clinicians treating them. Patient records will also be readily available, subject to the patient's consent, to all the relevant clinicians involved in their care which will substantially improve the co-ordination of the care provided.

8.12 Electronic patient records, whilst conforming to the requirements of security and confidentiality, will act as the basic building block for the other information the NHS needs in order to monitor quality. Information in them can be:

- used to support multi-disciplinary clinical audit at a local level;

- linked to other data about outcomes e.g. Office for National Statistics (ONS) death certificates, to provide timely and accurate information about the safety and quality of care provided by clinical teams and institutions;

- linked to ONS and other data to provide statistics for the routine surveillance and monitoring of mortality rates to provide an early warning of developing problems; and

- aggregated to provide management and performance assessment information.

8.13 Whilst electronic patient records will bring clear benefits, it will be several years before we will see them in place. In the meantime we are developing a range of initiatives to make better use of routinely collected data.

Hospital Episode Statistics (HES) data

Recommendation 150

The Hospital Episode Statistics database should be supported as a major national resource which can be used reliably, with care, to undertake the monitoring of a range of healthcare outcomes.

8.14 The Kennedy Report recommended that we should make better use of HES data. These data comprise basic information about clinical diagnosis and discharge or death. They do not contain the necessary clinical details to make full allowance for case mix or severity of illness and so cannot be used to produce absolute measures of quality. They are however a useful screening tool to help identify areas of concern where further exploration of the quality of care may be needed. We are working on:

- improving HES so that:
  - analysis can readily make use of links between different spells of care for the same patient to provide patient based rather than episode based views of care;
  - a wider range of measures of data quality is available and used as part of data use and feedback to the NHS;
  - the system has the capacity to be expanded in the future to cover outpatients, accident and emergency care, and private sector care to provide a fuller picture of the care pathway and the context of inpatient treatment; and
  - the system contains the necessary data items to provide meaningful analysis of the work of consultant teams. (Whilst data are held on consultant teams at present more work is required to produce robust analyses at this level).

- improving its value through linkage to ONS mortality data to allow better tracking of clinical outcomes;

- developing statistical methods to allow us to use routine data as part of a surveillance programme to identify potential problem areas; and

- developing a range of indicators, including the measurement of significant events, which can be used to identify potential problem areas in clinical quality.

Performance indicators

Recommendations 153, 155

Recommendation 153

At national level, the indicators of performance should be comprehensible to the public as well as to healthcare professionals. They should be fewer and of high quality, rather than numerous but of questionable or variable quality.

Recommendation 155

Patients and the public must be able to obtain information as to the relative performance of the trust and the services and consultant units within the trust.

115

The Department of Health's Response to the Report of the Public Inquiry into children's heart surgery at the Bristol Royal Infirmary 1984-1995

8.15   The publication *A Commitment to Quality, a Quest for Excellence* pledged us to work towards the provision of valid, reliable, up to date information on the quality of health services. Performance ratings were published for all acute NHS Trusts last year covering performance against the nine key targets and twelve other measures of performance. This work will be further refined and taken over by the Office for Information on Health Care Performance in due course. The Department, with the support of the BMA, wrote to NHS consultants in December 2001, telling them of its intention to use available data to publish performance information at consultant team level. We will work with the medical profession to improve local data collection.

National clinical audit

8.16   Although we recognise the need to focus on a few priorities and high level targets, health care is complex and to provide a rounded view of performance, indicators need to be available on specific services as well as on generic standards. For this reason we are developing with the relevant professional bodies a series of high quality national clinical audits that will enable the production of risk adjusted data about the quality of care for a range of important conditions.

8.17   High quality information is important if patients are to be able to make properly informed choices. We have been working with the Royal Colleges, the professional societies and patient representatives to build on the important work they have already undertaken in the field of clinical audit. Our aim is to publish high quality national information about the quality of care, which can be related to specific units and, in time, to specific consultants. We believe that this will be a valuable source of information for clinicians and patients alike. It will take time as well as commitment to make sure that the data are robust, that the clinicians are confident that it tells the correct story and that it informs rather than confuses the user. But we are committed to ensuring that within the foreseeable future all patients have access to data on the comparative performance of consultants and consultant teams.

8.18   We will begin this programme of national audit by developing programmes in each of the clinical priority areas in *The NHS Plan* - coronary heart disease, cancer, mental health and older people - and diabetes. We are working with the clinical professions to develop systems which produce national comparative data, risk adjusted where appropriate, so that individual clinicians, clinical teams, NHS Trusts and PCTs, the Department of Health, CHI and the public have the information they need to assess the quality of clinical care.

8.19 Substantial progress has been made in developing these systems with coronary heart disease in the vanguard. Paediatric cardiac surgeons have already developed national comparative data for peer review on the quality of their care and it will soon be possible to monitor the acute myocardial infarction 'call to needle time' target of the Coronary Heart Disease NSF as over 90% of hospitals are collecting the data required to produce comparative analyses.

8.20 For adult cardiac surgery, we have agreed a joint approach with the Society of Cardiothoracic Surgeons of Great Britain and Ireland to ensure the collection of reliable data on each and every patient undergoing a heart operation. Results from each of the cardiac centres have already been published and by April 2004 we will be able to publish 30 day mortality rates for the previous two years for every cardiac surgeon in England. From 2005 results will be published annually for each centre and for each cardiac surgeon on a rolling 3 year basis.

8.21 We recognise that differences in clinical practice and case mix can produce misleading comparative data. To avoid this we have agreed that the information for individual surgeons will be presented to show the clinical outcome for both routine cases and for their practice as a whole, reflecting the more complex cases undertaken.

8.22 This is just the first step to publishing more information on individual consultant outcomes. We are working with the medical profession to extend the number and range of specialties where information on both the consultant and the unit's comparative performance can be published on a regular basis. We will begin with the national clinical priority areas. In each case we will work closely with Royal Colleges and other professional groups to build on national audit work already in train.

8.23 Through the NHS Information Authority, the Department of Health is providing the information infrastructure to support the production of national comparative data in the NSF areas by co-ordinating the refinement and development of clinical audit datasets and databases so that data can be collated, analysed and fed back to clinicians and the other stakeholders. Central funding of just over £4m over two years has been provided through the Information for Health programme for this work - and we are exploring how best to support the service in capturing the data in advance of the widespread use of integrated clinical information systems.

8.24 We are developing national comparative data on:

- coronary heart disease:

- lung, breast and head and neck cancer;

- the implementation of the mental health Care Programme Approach; and

- for older people, stroke, continence and prescribing through snapshot audits.

8.25 Data on diabetes in adults will follow. In many cases, comparative data are already flowing to clinicians or will do so in 2002. However, additional work is required to produce complete national comparative data, ensure data quality, make links to related data (for example on mortality), to develop risk adjustment and to develop analyses for all stakeholders. A phased approach will be taken to developing the capacity to capture, collate, analyse and feed back data to clinicians in other areas. This work will become the responsibility of the Office for Information on Health Care Performance once it is established.

Local clinical audit

Recommendations 27, 143 - 145, 151

Recommendation 27

Patients should be referred to information relating to the performance of the trust, of the specialty and of the consultant unit (a consultant and the team of doctors who work under his or her supervision).

Recommendation 143

The process of clinical audit, which is now widely practised within trusts, should be at the core of a system of local monitoring of performance. Clinical audit should be multidisciplinary.

Recommendation 144

Clinical audit must be fully supported by trusts. They should ensure that healthcare professionals have access to the necessary time, facilities, advice and expertise in order to conduct audit effectively. All trusts should have a central clinical audit office which co-ordinates audit activity, provides advice and support for the audit process, and brings together the results of audit for the trust as a whole.

Recommendation 145

Clinical audit should be compulsory for all healthcare professionals providing clinical care and the requirement to participate in it should be included as part of the contract of employment.

Recommendation 151

Systems for clinical audit and for monitoring performance rely on accurate and complete data. Competent staff, trained in clinical coding, and supported in their work are required: the status, training and professional qualifications of clinical coding staff should be improved.

8.26 Under existing arrangements for clinical governance all NHS doctors are required to participate in audit programmes and from April 2001 it was made a contractual requirement. NHS Trusts are responsible for ensuring that their doctors meet this requirement and for providing the time and resources to enable multi-disciplinary clinical audit to take place. The clinical governance reviews undertaken by CHI monitor whether audit arrangements are in place, and NHS Trusts are required to report on their participation in and the impact of clinical audit activities in their annual clinical governance reports.

8.27 If patients are to be given good quality information about the risks and benefits of procedures they are to undergo, and clinicians are to have proper data on the outcome of different health care interventions we must have in place a strong system of locally based clinical audit. The purpose of audit is to assess the outcome of interventions and inform future practice and delivery of care.

8.28 The Kennedy Report recognises that systems for clinical audit rely on accurate and complete data, and for this we need competent, well trained and well supported staff. The NHS Information Authority is currently looking at the existing training infrastructure for clinical coders within the NHS to :

- provide recognition of the clinical coding professions;

- give organisations confidence in data quality; and

- help in the recruitment and assessment of clinical coding staff.

119

The Department of Health's Response to the Report of the Public Inquiry into children's heart surgery at the Bristol Royal Infirmary 1984-1995

Encouraging high quality data

> ### Recommendations 152, 156
>
> #### Recommendation 152
> **The system of incentives and penalties to encourage trusts to provide complete and validated data of a high quality to the national database should be reviewed. Any new system must include reports of each trust's performance in terms of the quality and timeliness of the submission of data. The systems within a trust for producing data of a high quality, and its performance in returning such data in a timely manner to the national database, should be taken into account in the process of validating and revalidating the trust.**
>
> #### Recommendation 156
> **As part of their Annual Reports, trust boards should be required to report on the extent of their compliance with the national clinical standards. These reports should be made public and be made available to CHI.**

8.29 The Kennedy Report recommends that the system of incentives and penalties to encourage NHS Trusts to provide high quality data should be reviewed. CHI has included scrutiny of the quality of data available to NHS Trusts as part of its regular reviews of clinical governance.

8.30 The Kennedy Report also recommends that as part of their annual reports, NHS Trust boards should be required to report on the extent of their compliance with national clinical standards. NHS Trusts are already required to report on progress on implementation of NSF and NICE guidelines as part of their annual clinical governance reports, which are public documents and made available to CHI.

Conclusion

8.31 Information is at the heart of everything we do in the NHS. Patients need good quality local data about their local NHS Trust - evidence of the patient experience, overall performance and, in time, the performance of the individual consultant responsible for their care. Clinicians and managers need information about what they are doing and how they are performing, not just as a NHS Trust, but in relation to others. We are already committed to a major investment programme to deliver the IT systems needed to support this information gathering; electronic patient records will be the key to unlocking and understanding the mass of data held throughout the system. We are committed to working with the professions to secure high quality, robust data about the relative clinical performance of specific units and plan in time to publish data in a way that is understandable to the clinician and the patient. As the Kennedy Report points out, the NHS already has a very wide range of data: our plans will allow us to use it effectively to inform individual choice, improve clinical care and support the modernisation of the NHS.

8.32 In responding to the Kennedy Report's recommendations on information, we will:

- publish over time data on the clinical performance of consultants and their units/teams for use by both clinicians and patients;

- by April 2004, publication of 30 day mortality rates for the previous two years for every cardiac surgeon in England. From April 2005 annual publication on a rolling three-year basis for each centre and for each cardiac surgeon;

- provide a co-ordinated approach to collecting data through the introduction of electronic patient records by 2005;

- make better use of HES data by linking to ONS mortality data from April 2002;

- publish 'star ratings' to compare the performance of NHS organisations against national targets – through the CHI Office of Information on Health Care Performance later in the year;

- undertake national audits in each of the clinical priority areas of *The NHS Plan*;

- set up a directory of clinical audit databases from 2002; and

- strengthen and support the clinical coding function.

INVOLVING PATIENTS AND THE PUBLIC IN HEALTH CARE

The NHS Plan sets out the Government's vision for a patient centred NHS. We want to move away from the system described in the Kennedy Report where there was little openness and where patients and others were kept at arm's length. Changing the culture will take time, but the reforms which are described below show how we are embedding the principles underpinning public and patient empowerment which Professor Kennedy set out in his report, into the health service which will help to ensure that the public, patients and their carers can influence the delivery of care at every level of the NHS.

Recommendation 157 and 165

Recommendation 157

The involvement of the public in the NHS must be embedded in its structures: the perspectives of patients and of the public must be heard and taken into account wherever decisions affecting the provision of healthcare are made.

Recommendation 165

The involvement of the public, particularly of patients, should not be limited to the representatives of patients' groups, or to those representing the interests of patients with a particular illness or condition; the NHS Modernisation Agency should advise the NHS on how to achieve the widest possible involvement of patients and the public in the NHS at local level.

9.1 We accept the principles outlined in the Kennedy Report that there should be greater openness and that patients should be equipped and supported to become genuine partners in their care. Current structures relate to an outdated model whereby patients, carers and their representatives campaign to be heard from outside the NHS. It is our aim to ensure that, where appropriate, the voices of citizens, patients and their carers are on the inside, influencing every level of the service. This is an ambition we share with the Kennedy Report, which emphasised:

> ...the priority for involving the public should be that their interests are embedded into all organisations and institutions concerned with quality of performance in the NHS: in other words, the public should be 'on the inside' rather than represented by some body 'on the outside'.

9.2   Transforming the NHS into a modern patient focused service is not primarily about extra investment or far reaching structural reforms. It means changing the culture and the way the NHS works, so that listening to, and acting on, the views of the people who use it becomes the norm and people are helped and encouraged to make their views known.

9.3   Patient Advice and Liaison Services (PALS) will be expected to work across organisational boundaries. We know that patients will often use many organisations as they progress through the patient journey. PALS will operate within a local network to provide support to patients and their carers as they pass from one organisation to another to ensure that patients' concerns are picked up and dealt with in the most appropriate way for each patient.

9.4   We already have 100 Pathfinder PALS and from April 2002 PALS will be in place in every NHS Trust and PCT in England, to provide information to patients, their carers and families and to help them resolve problems and concerns on the spot before they become more serious. PALS will also provide help by putting people in touch with specialist advocacy services, including independent advocacy and support to make a complaint.

9.5   The Health and Social Care Act 2001 puts in place the building blocks for our patient empowerment agenda. It enshrines in law:

- new powers for local government Overview and Scrutiny Committees to scrutinise the NHS;

- a new duty on the NHS to involve the public in the planning and development of services, and in major decisions; and

- a new duty on the Secretary of State to make independent advocacy services available to people wishing to make a complaint against the NHS.

9.6   But we also want patients and the public to have a greater say in the way local organisation and services are run. The NHS Reform and Health Care Professions Bill sets out our plans for:

- Patients' Forums in every PCT and NHS Trust in England; and

- a new national patients' body, the Commission for Patient and Public Involvement in Health, to set standards and provide training and guidance and monitor services from the patient's perspective. The Commission will also act as a local resource to build capacity within communities for engagement and involvement helping existing networks, and bring together the Patients' Forums in an area to provide them with a means of networking and sharing local experiences.

Patient Advice and Liaison Services (PALS)

Recommendations 29, 30, 32, 166

Recommendation 29

NHS trusts and primary care trusts must have systems which ensure that patients know where and to whom to go when they need further information or explanation.

Recommendation 30

We endorse the initiative in *'The NHS Plan'* to establish a Patient Advocacy and Liaison Service in every NHS trust and primary care trust. The establishment of this service should be implemented in full as quickly as possible. Once established, patient advocacy and liaison services must be given secure funding to enable them to provide an effective service to patients.

Recommendation 32

So as to provide for patients an effective, efficient and seamless information and advocacy service, consideration should be given to how the various patient advocacy and liaison services in a given geographical area could most effectively collaborate, including in relation to the provision of information for patients and the public.

Recommendation 166

Primary care trusts (and groups), given their capacity to influence the quality of care in hospitals, must involve patients and the public, for example through each PCG/T's Patient and Advocacy Liaison Service. They must make efforts systematically to gather views and feedback from patients. They must pay particular attention to involving their local community in decision-making about the commissioning of hospital services.

9.7 PALS will be a key source of information and feedback for the NHS Trust, PCT and the local Patients' Forum and will act as an early warning system, detecting, reporting and, where possible, resolving potential major problems before they escalate. PALS will send anonymised reports to the local Patients' Forum and to the NHS Trust and PCT about their work and action taken, identifying gaps in the system and areas for NHS staff training and development. The annual Patient Prospectus (see paragraph 9.11) will include information about changes that have been made as a result of PALS' work.

Patients' Forums

Recommendations 161 - 164

Recommendation 161

Proposals to establish Patients' Forums and Patients' Councils must allow for the involvement of the wider public and not be limited only to patients or to patients' groups. They must be seen as an addition to the process of involving patients and the public in the activities of the NHS, rather than as a substitute for it.

Recommendation 162

The mechanisms for the involvement of the public in the NHS should be routinely evaluated. These mechanisms should draw on the evidence of what works.

Recommendation 163

The process of public involvement must be properly supported, through for example, the provision of training and guidance.

Recommendation 164

Financial resources must be made available to enable members of the public to become involved in NHS organisations: this should include provision for payments to cover, for example, the costs of childcare, or loss of earnings.

9.8 We propose that the core remit of the Patients' Forum will be to find out what patients and carers think about the services they use, to monitor the quality of local services from the patient perspective, and to work with local NHS Trusts and PCTs to bring about improvements. They would be statutory independent bodies made up of patients and others from the local community, with extensive powers to inspect all aspects of the work of NHS Trusts and PCTs. They would elect one of their members on to the NHS Trust/PCT board, so allowing patients to elect a representative to the key decision making body of every local NHS organisation for the first time. They would be pivotal for people who use the services to become involved and have a real say in the way their local NHS is run. They would directly influence the quality and shape of services, with the goal of making the local NHS more responsive to what local patients actually want. Expenses will be paid to those who volunteer for Patients' Forums and PALS.

9.9   In going about their work, Patients' Forums would be able to:

- inspect every service that NHS patients use, including primary care services, and go behind the scenes;

- make their reports about the views and concerns of patients available to key decision makers in the community including the local Overview and Scrutiny Committees and Local Strategic Partnerships;

- monitor PALS and bring to the attention of the NHS Trust and PCT cases where this service is under performing. Where the service does not improve they should be able to recommend that it is replaced;

- report adverse incidents to the NPSA;

- make reports and recommendations for improvement of services to the NHS Trust and PCT boards based on the experiences, ideas and needs of patients and the wider public; and

- contribute evidence to inform CHI inspections and Health Select Committee inquiries.

Patient surveys

> **Recommendation 28**
>
> **Patients must be given the opportunity to pass on views on the service which they have received: all parts of the NHS should routinely seek and act on feedback from patients as to their views of the service. In addition, formal, systematic structured surveys of patients' experience of their care (not merely satisfaction surveys) should be routinely conducted across the NHS and the results made public.**

9.10 The new patient survey programme is an important tool for making the NHS more responsive to patients, and provides a formal mechanism for collecting patients' views on the services they receive. Starting this year, every acute hospital NHS Trust will undertake a new patient survey programme to use local patients' views to improve the quality of patients' experiences. Information from the patient survey programme will be included within the performance rating system to be published this year.

Patient Prospectus

Recommendations 31, 159

Recommendation 31

Trusts and primary care trusts must have systems for publishing periodic reports on patients' views and suggestions, including information about the action taken in the light of them.

Recommendation 159

The processes for involving patients and the public in organisations in the NHS must be transparent and open to scrutiny: the annual report of every organisation in the NHS should include a section setting out how the public has been involved, and the effect of that involvement.

9.11 To demonstrate that the NHS is acting on information gained from patients and responding to patients' priorities, every NHS Trust and PCT will be required to publish, in a new Patient Prospectus, an annual account of the views received from patients and local standards set specifically to address shortfalls identified through the new patient survey. Through the Patient Prospectus, NHS Trusts and PCTs will demonstrate how the public has been involved and the effect of that involvement. The annual Patient Prospectus will therefore act as a vehicle for publishing local targets and standards, describing how they are measured, progress made against them and new priorities - identified by patients - for the next year. The information gathered will be based on the patients' perspective, patients will agree the information and the information will be written so that patients can understand.

NICE Citizens' Council

> **Recommendations 42, 105, 158**
>
> **Recommendation 42**
>
> **All the various bodies and organisations concerned with regulation, besides being independent of government, must involve and reflect the interests of patients, the public and healthcare professionals, as well as the NHS and government.**
>
> **Recommendation 105**
>
> **The need to involve the public in the various professional regulatory bodies applies as much to discipline as to all the other activities of these bodies.**
>
> **Recommendation 158**
>
> **Organisations which are not part of the NHS but have an impact on it, such as Royal Colleges, the GMC, the Nursing and Midwifery Council and the body responsible for regulating the professions allied to medicine, must involve the public in their decision-making processes, as they affect the provision of healthcare by the NHS.**

9.12   *The NHS Plan* sets out our commitment to create a Citizens' Council to advise NICE on the values inherent in its decisions and guidance on treatments. The Department of Health is currently working with NICE to develop a Council that is broadly representative of the English and Welsh populations. We will draw on the lessons learned by Citizens' Juries to ensure that members of the Council have enough time and information to deliberate on the questions and give their advice to NICE. We support the view that the bodies concerned with regulation should involve and reflect the interests of patients. We are looking to the GMC to make proposals for its future governance, which will reflect this. The new Nursing and Midwifery and Health Professions Councils and the Council for the Regulation of Health Care Professionals will reflect the interests of patients, the public and health care staff. The UKCC for Nursing and Midwifery and Health Visiting has already published a *Strategy for Public Involvement.* We would commend this approach to the other regulatory bodies. NICE, CHI, NPSA and NCAA all involve the public and patients in their work and decision making.

Commission for Patient and Public Involvement in Health (CPPIH)

Recommendation 160

The public's involvement in the NHS should particularly be focused on the development and planning of healthcare services and on the operation and delivery of healthcare services, including the regulation of safety and quality, the competence of healthcare professionals, and the protection of vulnerable groups.

9.13 The Commission for Patient and Public Involvement in Health will be a new national body for patients and will oversee the local structures for public and patient involvement. It will set standards and provide training and guidance for the new public and patient involvement mechanisms. It will:

- facilitate the effective operation of patient and public involvement and representation systems at local, regional and national level;

- identify and disseminate quality standards for the establishment, operation and evaluation of the public and patient involvement system;

- set criteria for this evaluation and make recommendations and reports to the Secretary of State on the outcome of this;

- inform, advise and support local public and patient involvement bodies;

- provide a national assessment of the performance of the public and patient involvement system; and

- report to other independent bodies, such as CHI and NPSA, data on matters relating to patient safety and welfare that emerge through the whole system of patient and public involvement.

In addition to these national functions the Commission will also undertake a set of functions at PCT level by a network of specialists. It is likely that there will be one team of specialists for each Strategic Health Authority area.

9.14 The key aim of these teams will be to engender and promote public involvement in the NHS – ensuring that as many people as possible have their say and are able to become involved. It will do this by training people who are interested and, where necessary, organise separate public involvement exercises so that community views are comprehensively reflected in local decisions that affect the health of communities. In addition:

- they will work alongside Patients' Forums helping them to undertake their functions;

- they will facilitate and co-ordinate the work of Patients' Forums across a wider area than just their own specific service responsibility area – picking up the patient's journey data and highlighting trends and issues across a health economy;

- they will provide administrative support to Patients' Forums in their area; and

- it will be possible for them to commission independent complaints advocacy services across an agreed geographical area.

Figure 2.   Greater Patient and Public Involvement

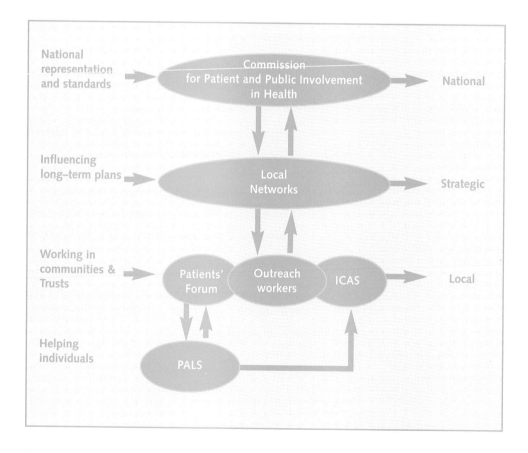

Conclusion

9.15 There are a number of initiatives in prospect which will set the foundation for a new approach to including the public and patients in the design, operation and delivery of health care. For the first time patients and the public will be fully supported in telling us their views; their views will be listened to and they will be influential in making key decisions about the shape of health care provision for the future and the way services are designed and delivered on a day to day basis. The strategy we have in place will genuinely place patients and the public at the very centre of what we do.

9.16 We will encourage the greater involvement of patients and the public in health care by:

- establishing Patient Advice and Liaison Services (PALS) in every NHS Trust and PCT from April 2002;

- establishing, through the NHS Reform and Health Care Professions Bill:
  - Patients' Forums in every PCT and NHS Trust in England to promote patient and carer interests in the NHS, by representing their views to NHS Trusts and PCTs and sitting on Trust boards, and by scrutinising local services; and
  - the Commission for Patient and Public Involvement in Health, to set standards and provide training and guidance and build capacity within local communities for greater community involvement;

- introducing the patient survey programme from 2001 to inform local decision making;

- requiring every NHS Trust and PCT to publish an annual Patient Prospectus to demonstrate how the public have been involved and the effect of that involvement; and

- establishing a Citizens' Council to advise NICE on the values inherent in its decisions and guidance on treatments.

131

The Department of Health's Response to the Report of the Public Inquiry into children's heart surgery at the Bristol Royal Infirmary 1984-1995

Chapter 10

LOOKING TO THE FUTURE

10.1 The Report of the BRI Inquiry has set us a challenging task. In discovering what happened at Bristol, the Report describes 'a tragedy born of high hopes and ambitions' and a service that had too high expectations. The challenge that faces us is to deliver a health service with high hopes and ambitions, but with the culture, the systems and the resources to deliver them.

10.2 The March 2000 Budget settlement means that the NHS will grow by 50% in cash terms or by more than a third in real terms in just 5 years. In addition we have recently announced a further billion pounds for health care across the UK for 2002/3. This step change in resources is being matched by a step change in reform. *The NHS Plan* sets out how we will deliver a health service fit for the twenty first century - delivering better health and faster, fairer and more convenient services. This Response details progress on this work, as well as the further action we propose to give reality to the spirit of the Kennedy Report.

10.3 Some of the recommendations of the Report will require planned investment over a number of years, others are about changing attitudes and approaches in the way we plan and deliver our services. Implementation of the Report will take time: transforming the NHS cannot be achieved overnight. We are committed to making change happen. The key tasks that face us are:

- putting patients at the centre of health care delivery;

- investing in staff;

- improving children's health care services;

- strengthening the regulation and inspection of health care;

- ensuring the safety of care; and

- including the public in decision making in the NHS.

10.4 The Kennedy Report is honest in recognising that the change it envisages will take time as well as resources. We have already said that *The NHS Plan* is a ten year programme. But we believe that our proposals to invest heavily in the workforce and the infrastructure are central to moving towards the vision of a modern, patient centred NHS. They are the key which will unlock the potential of the NHS to meet the challenges placed on it – not just increasing the number of procedures it can undertake – but to improving the quality of the patients' experience and the way they experience the delivery of all aspects of care.

10.5 Culture change is difficult. It will take time, commitment and energy. We are committed to delivering a high quality modern health service. We are investing and building a health service where patients and the public are genuinely involved in decision making; where staff work in multi-disciplinary teams to deliver care that genuinely reflects the needs of the patient; where staff can aspire to give of their best and are genuinely supported in so doing; and above all where there is an open, honest culture to provide the best of modern health care in a safe environment. Clinical governance provides the framework to ensure that every local NHS organisation demonstrates a commitment to quality, the ability to reflect on past practice and learn from mistakes. It ensures the active involvement of patients, users and carers and provides support for continuous quality improvement across the whole of the NHS.

10.6 The Kennedy Report has set us a challenge. In framing its recommendations the Inquiry Panel aimed to build a bridge between the lessons of the past and the NHS of the future, so Bristol will be remembered not merely as a synonym for tragedy but also as a turning point for the NHS. It is for us – all of us - to ensure that this is indeed the case.

RECOMMENDATIONS AND RESPONSES

Recommendation 1

In a patient-centred healthcare service patients must be involved, wherever possible, in decisions about their treatment and care.

We agree. As promised in *The NHS Plan*, we have introduced a 'good practice in consent' initiative to ensure patients are able to be involved in their own health care decisions. The Reference Guide sets out the current legal position; guidance for patients on consent is available throughout the NHS; a model consent policy and model consent forms were issued in November 2001 for implementation throughout the NHS. Implementation will be monitored through clinical governance, the Clinical Negligence Scheme for Trusts, the Controls Assurance Framework and will be subject to inspection by CHI.

Recommendation 2

The education and training of all healthcare professionals should be imbued with the idea of partnership between the healthcare professional and the patient.

We agree. *The NHS Plan* stresses the importance of communicating well with patients and their families – this will be reflected in education and training programmes as part of basic training and as part of continuing professional development.

Recommendation 3

The notion of partnership between the healthcare professional and the patient, whereby the patient and the professional meet as equals with different expertise, must be adopted by healthcare professionals in all parts of the NHS, including healthcare professionals in hospitals.

We agree. The new core curriculum which will be in place by 2002 will help to break down traditional barriers between health professionals and patients. The Expert Patient Programme is also being introduced to support patients in this relationship. From 2002, pilot sites in PCTs and PCGs will cover between 50,000 and 75,000 people with long-term conditions and there will be full implementation from 2004 covering between 300,000 - 450,000 people.

Information about treatment and care should be given in a variety of forms, be given in stages and be reinforced over time.

We agree. The model consent policy requires NHS organisations to make good quality up to date information available to patients in a variety of forms and makes it clear that consent is a continuing process, not a one-off event. (See response to recommendation 1 above).

Information should be tailored to the needs, circumstances and wishes of the individual.

We agree. From April 2003 information will be made available through the new National Knowledge Service in a number of languages and aimed at different levels of understanding. The NHS Modernisation Agency will play a role in identifying and sharing good practice.

Information should be based on the current available evidence and include a summary of the evidence and data, in a form which is comprehensible to patients.

We agree. The new National Knowledge Service for the NHS will provide a framework for identifying and meeting the needs for knowledge to support patient care.

Various modes of conveying information, whether leaflets, tapes, videos or CDs, should be regularly updated, and developed and piloted with the help of patients.

We agree. Wider access to information is being developed through a range of technologies, including NHS Direct Information Points and Information channels on bedside TVs. Bedside phones and TVs will be available in every major hospital by December 2003.

The NHS Modernisation Agency should make the improvement of the quality of information for patients a priority. In relation to the content and the dissemination of information for patients, the Agency should identify and promote good practice throughout the NHS. It should establish a system for accrediting materials intended to inform patients.

We agree. Promoting good practice throughout the NHS in relation to quality of information for patients is an integral part of all NHS Modernisation Agency programmes.

Recommendation 9

The public should receive guidance on those sources of information about health and healthcare on the Internet which are reliable and of good quality: a kitemarking system should be developed.

We agree. The new National Knowledge Service will integrate existing systems e.g. DH websites, NHS Direct, National Electronic Library for Health. NHS Direct Online is already accrediting some material and we plan to extend this further from 2003.

Recommendation 10

Tape-recording facilities should be provided by the NHS to enable patients, should they so wish, to make a tape recording of a discussion with a healthcare professional when a diagnosis, course of treatment, or prognosis is being discussed.

We reject this proposal, as we believe it could undermine the relationship of trust between the patient and health care professional.

Recommendation 11

Patients should always be given the opportunity and time to ask questions about what they are told, to seek clarification and to ask for more information. It must be the responsibility of employers in the NHS to ensure that the working arrangements of healthcare professionals allow for this, not least that they have the necessary time.

We agree. The new model consent forms make clear that patients should be encouraged to ask questions and raise any concerns that they may have. We are also investing significant new resources to increase the number of doctors, nurses and therapists, which will contribute to quality improvement in the NHS and the ability to ensure patients fully understand what is proposed.

By 2004 there will be:

- 7,500 more consultants

- 2,000 more GPs

- 20,000 more nurses

- 6,500 more therapists.

Recommendation 12

Patients must be given such information as enables them to participate in their care.

We agree. The steps outlined above in response to recommendations 1-11 will help to ensure patients have access to information while receiving care. In addition the new guidance on consent makes clear that patients must have sufficient information on any proposed procedure before their consent to treatment is sought.

Recommendations 13 and 16

Before embarking on any procedure, patients should be given an explanation of what is going to happen and, after the procedure, should have the opportunity to review what has happened.

Patients should be given the sense of freedom to indicate when they do not want any (or more) information: this requires skill and understanding from healthcare professionals.

We agree. Communicating well with patients means listening and responding to the needs of patients in terms of information which they actually want. This is a key part of our initiative to improve communications within the NHS and we will ensure that it is built into training at all levels.

Recommendations 14, 17 and 18

Patients should be supported in dealing with the additional anxiety sometimes created by greater knowledge.

Patients should receive a copy of any letter written about their care or treatment by one healthcare professional to another.

Parents of those too young to take decisions for themselves should receive a copy of any letter written by one healthcare professional to another about their child's treatment or care.

We agree. Health care staff are trained to respond to the emotional and spiritual needs of their patients and provide the support they need. A working group which includes patients, doctors, nurses, hospital records management staff and representatives of professionals organisations, was set up in July 2001 to produce guidelines on copying clinicians' letters to patients. It will also address how best to support patients in dealing with the anxiety sometimes caused by greater knowledge and set out arrangements whereby parents will receive copies of letters when children are too young to receive the information themselves. The Working Group will produce its guidelines by the summer of 2002.

137

The Department of Health's Response to the Report of the Public Inquiry into children's heart surgery at the Bristol Royal Infirmary 1984-1995

Recommendation 15

Patients should be told that they may have another person of their choosing present when receiving information about a diagnosis or a procedure.

We agree. The patient's leaflet *Consent – what you have a right to expect* (published in July 2001) encourages patients to take someone with them to a consultation, if they wish.

Recommendation 19

Healthcare professionals responsible for the care of any particular patient must communicate effectively with each other. The aim must be to avoid giving the patient conflicting advice and information.

We agree. Our communications initiative will ensure patients are at the centre of care and the focus of team working and inter-professional care. Health care professionals will develop these skills through joint learning and working at all levels of the NHS.

Recommendation 20

The provision of counselling and support should be regarded as an integral part of a patient's care. All hospital trusts should have a well-developed system and a well-trained group of professionals whose task it is to provide this type of support and to make links to the various other forms of support (such as that provided by voluntary or social services) which patients may need.

We agree. PALS will provide an accessible service to patients and their families, providing information and support on all aspects of Trust services including access to specialist counselling. PALs will be introduced into every NHS Trust and PCT from April 2002.

Recommendation 21

Every trust should have a professional bereavement service. (We also reiterate what was recommended in the Inquiry's Interim Report: 'Recommendation 13: As hospitals develop websites, a domain should be created concerned with bereavement in which all the relevant information concerning post-mortems can be set out in an appropriate manner.')

We agree. The Department is currently mapping the quality and quantity of bereavement services to determine where specific improvements are needed. This work is nearing completion and will inform the need for change. Separately, work is progressing to develop a Code of Practice on communicating with families about post-mortems – this will include setting up a bereavement section on NHS Trust websites. The Code of Practice has been issued for consultation in January 2002. A Department of Health website on bereavement is already in place (www.doh.gov.uk/bereavement).

Recommendation 22

Voluntary organisations which provide care and support to patients and carers in the NHS (such as through telephone helplines, the provision of information and the organisation of self-help groups) play a very important role. Groups which meet the appropriate standards as laid down by the NHS should receive appropriate funding from the state for the contribution they make to the NHS.

We agree. Voluntary organisations can already be funded to provide such services as an alternative to the NHS providing the services itself.

Recommendation 23

We note and endorse the recent statement on consent produced by the DoH: *'Reference guide to consent for examination or treatment'*, 2001. It should inform the practice of all healthcare professionals in the NHS and be introduced into practice in all trusts.

We agree. The model consent policy requires NHS organisations to consider the procedural factors which will effect how patients actually experience the consent process, e.g. time at which consent sought, availability of written information. The model consent policy was issued in November 2001.

Recommendation 24

The process of informing the patient, and obtaining consent to a course of treatment, should be regarded as a process and not a one-off event consisting of obtaining a patient's signature on a form.

We agree. Both the Reference Guide and the model consent policy make very clear that consent is a process – the signing of a consent form (where appropriate) is only the end point.

Recommendation 25

The process of consent should apply not only to surgical procedures but to all clinical procedures and examinations which involve any form of touching. This must not mean more forms: it means more communication.

We agree. Both the Reference Guide and the model consent policy make very clear that consent should always be sought before any kind of personal care or treatment is offered.

139

The Department of Health's Response to the Report of the Public Inquiry into children's heart surgery at the Bristol Royal Infirmary 1984-1995

Recommendation 26

As part of the process of obtaining consent, except when they have indicated otherwise, patients should be given sufficient information about what is to take place, the risks, uncertainties, and possible negative consequences of the proposed treatment, about any alternatives and about the likely outcome, to enable them to make a choice about how to proceed.

We agree. The new model consent forms make clear that patients should be informed about benefits, risks, what the treatment will involve and about alternative treatments if available. Model forms were issued in November 2001. Controls Assurance, the Clinical Negligence Scheme for Trusts and clinical governance and CHI inspections should ensure that they are used in all Trusts.

Recommendation 27

Patients should be referred to information relating to the performance of the trust, of the specialty and of the consultant unit (a consultant and the team of doctors who work under his or her supervision).

We agree. A range of new developments is contributing to the collection of better information about the performance of NHS Trusts. A wider range of information is now available in a form which is more readily understood by members of the public. This information includes the annual publication of performance indicators for all acute Trusts, the clinical governance reviews undertaken by CHI as part of their programme of inspection, and the publication of improved clinical indicators.

We have collaborated with 'Dr Foster' on a number of initiatives including their 'Good Hospital' and 'Good Consultant Guides', and we are working with the Royal Colleges to make better and more systematic use of clinical audit data, with a view to publication, in time, of consultant specific data.

Recommendation 28

Patients must be given the opportunity to pass on views on the service which they have received: all parts of the NHS should routinely seek and act on feedback from patients as to their views of the service. In addition, formal, systematic structured surveys of patients' experience of their care (not merely satisfaction surveys) should be routinely conducted across the NHS and the results made public.

We agree. Starting this year, every acute hospital Trust will undertake an annual patient survey. We have introduced legislation to establish Patients' Forums in every NHS Trust and PCT to be in place by April 2003. The Forum will provide external scrutiny and examine the results from the patient survey and make recommendations for service improvements to the Trust board.

Recommendation 29

NHS trusts and primary care trusts must have systems which ensure that patients know where and to whom to go when they need further information or explanation.

We agree. From April 2002 every NHS Trust and PCT will have a PALS to help and advise patients, their carers and families.

Recommendation 30

We endorse the initiative in *'The NHS Plan'* to establish a Patient Advocacy and Liaison Service in every NHS trust and primary care trust. The establishment of this service should be implemented in full as quickly as possible. Once established, patient advocacy and liaison services must be given secure funding to enable them to provide an effective service to patients.

We agree. £10 million was allocated in 2001/2 to establish 100 'Pathfinder' PALS. From April 2002 PALS will be in place in every Trust. Their future funding will be through normal Trust allocations.

Recommendation 31

Trusts and primary care trusts must have systems for publishing periodic reports on patients' views and suggestions, including information about the action taken in the light of them.

We agree. From 2002/3 every Trust should publish in a new Patient Prospectus, an annual account of patients' views and local standards set specifically to address shortfalls and identified through the new patient survey.

Recommendation 32

So as to provide for patients an effective, efficient and seamless information and advocacy service, consideration should be given to how the various patient advocacy and liaison services in a given geographical area could most effectively collaborate, including in relation to the provision of information for patients and the public.

We agree. PCT PALS will be expected to act as lead PALS, co-ordinating effective collaboration across their areas.

Recommendations 33 and 34

A duty of candour, meaning a duty to tell a patient if adverse events have occurred, must be recognised as owed by all those working in the NHS to patients.

The Department of Health's Response to the Report of the Public Inquiry into children's heart surgery at the Bristol Royal Infirmary 1984-1995

When things go wrong, patients are entitled to receive an acknowledgement, an explanation and an apology.

We agree. Patients are entitled to a full explanation and apology when something goes wrong whether or not they wish to make a complaint. Under the current complaints procedure, acknowledgements should be made within 2 days; full investigations and resolution should be made within 20 working days (10 days in primary care) and an explanation and/or an apology offered as appropriate. The broader implications for clinical negligence legislation will be addressed in the CMO's work on clinical negligence, leading to a White Paper early in 2002.

Recommendation 35

There should be a clear system, in the form of a 'one-stop shop' in every trust, for addressing the concerns of a patient about the care provided by, or the conduct of, a healthcare professional.

We agree. PALS will be in place by April 2002 in every NHS Trust to help and advise patients to resolve immediate concerns or problems about the care provided or the conduct of a health care professional.

Recommendation 36

Complaints should be dealt with swiftly and thoroughly, keeping the patient (and carer) informed. There should be a strong independent element, not part of the trust's management or board, in any body considering serious complaints which require formal investigation. An independent advocacy service should be established to assist patients (and carers).

(See also response to Recommendation 34). We agree in part. We are reviewing the current NHS Complaints System. The review will be completed by the end of 2002. As part of the review we will be looking at strengthening the independent review stage of the existing complaints system. PALS will be available to assist patients through the complaints process.

Recommendation 37

There should be an urgent review of the system for providing compensation to those who suffer harm arising out of medical care. The review should be concerned with the introduction of an administrative system for responding promptly to patients' needs in place of the current system of clinical negligence and should take account of other administrative systems for meeting the financial needs of the public.

We agree. We have already announced plans to produce a White Paper early in 2002, discussing options for reform to the system for dealing with clinical negligence claims.

Recommendation 38

The DoH's roles in relation to the NHS must in future be made explicit. The DoH should have two roles. It should be the headquarters of the NHS. It should also establish an independent framework of regulation which will assure the quality of the care provided in and funded by the NHS, and the competence of healthcare professionals.

We agree. The Department of Health in supporting the Secretary of State will be responsible for setting the overall direction for the NHS, securing its funding, determining major investments and ensuring that there are appropriate arrangements in place for its management, standard setting, inspection, improvement and accountability. It will be responsible for ensuring that the various bodies responsible for these different functions work together to provide a consistent framework of high delivery health improvement and health care for the population.

Recommendation 39

The framework of regulation must consist of two overarching organisations, independent of government, which bring together the various bodies which regulate healthcare. A Council for the Quality of Healthcare should be created to bring together those bodies which regulate healthcare standards and institutions (including for example, the Commission for Health Improvement (CHI), the National Institute for Clinical Excellence (NICE) and the proposed National Patient Safety Agency). A Council for the Regulation of Healthcare Professionals should be created to bring together those bodies which regulate healthcare professionals (including, for example, the General Medical Council (GMC) and the Nursing and Midwifery Council); in effect, this is the body currently referred to in 'The NHS Plan' as the Council of Healthcare Regulators. These overarching organisations must ensure that there is an integrated and co-ordinated approach to setting standards, monitoring performance, and inspection and validation. Issues of overlap and of gaps between the various bodies must be addressed and resolved.

We agree. Proposals for the creation of the Council for the Regulation of Health Care Professionals were published for consultation in August 2001. They are designed to replace the current fragmented arrangements and to lead to more effective co-ordination and clearer accountability mechanisms. We plan to legislate to effect the changes in the NHS Reform and Health Care Professions Bill.

143

The Department of Health's Response to the Report of the Public Inquiry into children's heart surgery at the Bristol Royal Infirmary 1984-1995

Recommendation 40

The two Councils should be independent of government and report both to the DoH and to Parliament. There should be close collaboration between the two Councils. The DoH should establish and fund the Councils and set their strategic framework, and thereafter periodically review them.

We agree in principle. We will establish and fund a new administrative Council for Quality of Health Care in 2002 to ensure co-ordination between the Council for the Regulation of Health Care Professionals and other organisations with an interest in service quality, including NICE, CHI, NCAA and the NPSA. This will be at arm's length from the Department of Health. The Council for the Regulation of Health Care Professionals will be independent and report to Parliament.

Recommendation 41

The various bodies whose purpose it is to assure the quality of care in the NHS (for example, CHI and NICE) and the competence of healthcare professionals (for example, the GMC and the Nursing and Midwifery Council) must themselves be independent of and at arm's-length from the DoH.

We agree. Those bodies whose purpose it is to assure quality of care and health care professional regulatory bodies should remain independent and at arm's length from the Department of Health. The status of CHI as a non departmental public body and NICE as a Special Health Authority will remain unchanged.

Recommendation 42

All the various bodies and organisations concerned with regulation, besides being independent of government, must involve and reflect the interests of patients, the public and healthcare professionals, as well as the NHS and government.

We agree. Proposals for the new Nursing and Midwifery and Health Professions Councils and reform of the GMC include arrangements for reflecting the interests of patients, the public and health care professionals. We are encouraging all regulatory bodies to develop similar arrangements.

Recommendation 43

The contractual relationship between trusts and consultants should be redefined. The trust must provide the consultant with the time, space and the necessary tools to do the job. Consultants must accept that the time spent in the hospital and what they do in that time must be explicitly set out.

We agree. Under the Government's proposals for the new consultant contract, all consultants' job plans will explicitly set out how their working time should be organised and what support the Trust should provide.

Recommendation 44

The system of Distinction Awards for hospital consultants should be examined to determine whether it could be used to provide greater incentives than exist at present for providing good quality of care to patients. The possibility of its extension to include junior hospital doctors should be explored.

We agree. The new NHS Clinical Excellence Awards will reward those who make the biggest contribution to delivering and improving health services in terms of leadership and clinical excellence.

Recommendation 45

The doctors' Code of Professional Practice, as set down in the GMC's *'Good Medical Practice'*, should be incorporated into the contract of employment between doctors and trusts. In the case of GPs, the terms of service should be amended to incorporate the Code.

We reject. The standard documentation for consultants' appraisal – a contractual requirement from April 2001 – already explicitly includes the headings set out in the GMC's *Good Medical Practice*. The same principles will apply to other NHS doctors including GPs where appraisal is under negotiation.

Recommendation 46

The relevant codes of practice for nurses, for professions allied to medicine and for managers should be incorporated into their contracts of employment with hospital trusts or primary care trusts.

We agree in principle. Contracts of employment for health care professionals are already based on the premise that they are properly registered with their regulatory body. Many contracts include this specific provision but it is implicit in all contracts of employment.

Recommendation 47

Trusts should be able to deal as employers with breaches of the relevant professional code by a healthcare professional, independently of any action which the relevant professional body may take.

We agree in principle. We expect that local employers take into account professional codes of practice in their local codes of conduct.

Recommendation 48

The security of tenure of the chief executive and senior managers of trusts should be on a par with that of other senior professionals in the NHS.

We agree in principle and are considering this issue in more detail as part of work to develop a new framework for senior managers' contracts.

Recommendation 49

The criteria and process for selection of the executive directors of a trust board must be open and transparent. Appointments should be made on the basis of ability and not on the basis of seniority.

We agree. The appointment procedures for executive directors are rigorous – guidance was issued in December 1997 (EL (97) 84).

Recommendation 50

The NHS Leadership Centre, in conjunction with trusts, should develop programmes of training and support for clinicians and others who seek to become executive directors.

We agree. An executive director development programme will commence in January 2002.

Recommendation 51

As recommended in *'The NHS Plan'*, there should be an NHS Appointments Commission responsible for the appointment of non-executive directors of NHS trusts, health authorities and primary care trusts.

We agree. The NHS Appointments Commission was established on 1 April 2001.

Recommendation 52

Newly appointed non-executive directors of trusts, health authorities and primary care trusts should receive a programme of induction: this should refer to the principles and values of the NHS and their duties and responsibilities with regard to the quality of care provided by the trust. This programme should be provided through the NHS Leadership Centre.

We agree. An induction guide for chairs and non-executive directors is being developed by the NHS Leadership Centre and the NHS Appointments Commission. It will be published in January 2002.

Recommendation 53

A standard job description should be developed by the NHS for non-executive directors, as proposed in *'The NHS Plan'*.

We agree. A standard description for chairmen and non-executive directors has been developed and is used in the recruitment of all chairs and non-executives.

Recommendation 54

Throughout their period of tenure, non-executive directors should be provided with training, support and advice organised and co-ordinated through the NHS Leadership Centre.

We agree. The NHS Leadership Centre will continue working with Regional Commissioners in the design of development initiatives for non-executive directors.

Recommendation 55

The Chairs of trust boards should have a source of independent advice (or mentor) during their period of office, drawn from a pool of experts assembled by the NHS Leadership Centre.

We agree. The NHS Leadership Centre will act as "broker" in matching chairs of Trust boards with mentors or sources of independent advice.

Recommendation 56

Arrangements should be in place in the standing orders of trust boards to provide for proper continuity in the management of the trust's affairs in the period between the cessation of the Chair's term of office and the commencement of that of a successor.

We agree. The NHS Appointments Commission will ensure that there is rarely a gap between the retirement of a chairman and appointment of a successor.

Recommendation 57

Greater priority than at present should be given to non-clinical aspects of care in six key areas in the education, training and continuing professional development of healthcare professionals:

- **skills in communicating with patients and with colleagues;**

147

The Department of Health's Response to the Report of the Public Inquiry into children's heart surgery at the Bristol Royal Infirmary 1984-1995

- education about the principles and organisation of the NHS, and about how care is managed, and the skills required for management;

- the development of teamwork;

- shared learning across professional boundaries;

- clinical audit and reflective practice; and

- leadership.

We agree. We are working with regulatory and professional bodies and educators to ensure that from 2002 these core skills are including in all NHS funded professional programmes and clinical undergraduate training.

Recommendation 58

Competence in non-clinical aspects of caring for patients should be formally assessed as part of the process of obtaining an initial professional qualification, whether as a doctor, a nurse or some other healthcare professional.

We agree. The non-clinical aspects of care are already a core part of the training of health professionals. We are currently working with the professions and educationalists to strengthen non-clinical aspects of care as part of a common learning approach across professions.

Recommendation 59

Education in communication skills must be an essential part of the education of all healthcare professionals. Communication skills include the ability to engage with patients on an emotional level to listen, to assess how much information a patient wants to know, and to convey information with clarity and sympathy.

We agree. Education in communication skills is a core feature of professional training. We have now begun a major new communications skills initiative which will encompass all NHS staff and reflect the values set out in *The NHS Plan.*

Recommendations 60 and 61

Communication skills must also include the ability to engage with and respect the views of fellow healthcare professionals.

The education, training and Continuing Professional Development (CPD) of all healthcare professionals should include joint courses between the professions.

We agree. Ability to engage with and respect fellow health professionals is crucial. Common learning will be included at all stages of education, training and CPD. Leading edge sites are being supported from 2001/02 and we will evaluate them.

Recommendation 62

There should be more opportunities than at present for multi-professional teams to learn, train and develop together.

We agree. More opportunities for multi-professional teams to train together are emerging as the common learning programme is rolled out.

Recommendation 63

All those preparing for a career in clinical care should receive some education in the management of healthcare, the health service and the skills required for management.

We agree. Education in management of health care and the health service and development of the management skills required, are included and assessed in all professional curricula. We will continue to work with professional bodies and education institutions to ensure that these important areas receive the prominence they require.

Recommendation 64

Greater opportunities should be created for managers and clinicians to 'shadow' one another for short periods to learn about their roles and work pressures.

We agree. The NHS Leadership Centre will ensure that managers and clinicians have more opportunities to learn about their respective roles and work pressures through the Lifelong Learning programme.

Recommendation 65

An early priority for the new NHS Leadership Centre should be to offer guidelines as to the leadership styles and practices which are acceptable and to be encouraged within the NHS, and those which are not.

We agree. A values and behaviours framework for leadership is in the final stages of development and will be distributed to all Trusts by the end of February 2002.

Recommendation 66

Steps should be taken to identify and train those within the NHS who have the potential to exercise leadership. There needs to be a sustained investment in developing leadership skills at all levels in the NHS.

We agree. Considerable investment in leadership development has been made and continues as new programmes are designed and delivered. By March 2002, 325 doctors will have attended leadership programmes and by November 2002, over 33,000 nurses and allied health professionals will have done so.

Recommendation 67

The NHS's investment in developing and funding programmes in leadership skills should be focused on supporting joint education and multi-professional training, open to nurses, doctors, managers and other healthcare professionals.

We agree. The new executive directors' development programme focuses on multi-professional roles for medical and nursing directors and interaction with general managers and finance colleagues.

Recommendation 68

The NHS Leadership Centre should be involved in all stages of the education, training and continuing development of all healthcare professionals.

We agree. The NHS Leadership Centre will work alongside Workforce Confederations and Higher Education colleagues to influence curriculum planning.

Recommendations 69 and 74

Regulation of healthcare professionals is not just about disciplinary matters. It should be understood as encapsulating all of the systems which combine to assure the competence of healthcare professionals: education, registration, training, CPD and revalidation as well as disciplinary matters.

It should be a priority for the Council for the Regulation of Healthcare Professionals to promote common curricula and shared learning across the professions.

We agree in part. We recognise that the regulatory bodies have considerable expertise and specialisation in the field of education, training and development. We agree that the new Council should be able to ensure that a single overarching view is taken of education, training and development. We do not agree that the new Council should be given powers to determine standards for education and admission to practise.

Recommendation 70

For *each* group of healthcare professionals (doctors, nurses and midwives, the professions allied to medicine, and managers) there should be one body charged with overseeing *all* aspects relating to the regulation of professional life: education, registration, training, CPD, revalidation and discipline. The bodies should be: for doctors, the GMC; for nurses and midwives, the new Nursing and Midwifery Council; for the professions allied to medicine, the re-formed professional body for those professions; and for senior healthcare managers, a new professional body.

We agree in part. The GMC and the new Nursing and Midwifery and Health Professional Councils will have a duty to work with other organisations including employers and educators. However, we do not agree that the GMC should act as the competent authority for medical training (see also response to Recommendation 81).

Recommendation 71

In addition, a single body should be charged with the overall co-ordination of the various professional bodies and with integrating the various systems of regulation. It should be called the Council for the Regulation of Healthcare Professionals. (In effect, this is the body currently proposed in *'The NHS Plan'*, and referred to as the Council of Healthcare Regulators.)

We agree. Proposals for a Council for the Regulation of Health Care Professionals were set out in a consultation document *Modernising Regulation in the Health Professions*, published in August 2001 and we have introduced legislation to give these effect.

Recommendation 72

The Council for the Regulation of Healthcare Professionals should be established as a matter of priority. It should have a statutory basis. It should report to Parliament. It should have a broadly-based membership, consisting of representatives of the bodies which regulate the various groups of healthcare professionals, of the NHS, and of the general public.

We agree. We propose that the Council for the Regulation of Health Care Professionals should be accountable to Parliament. We propose that the new Council should have 17 members: 1 nominee from each of the current 9 regulatory bodies and 10 members to represent patients, public and NHS interests; one of these appointed by each of the three devolved administrations and 7 by the Secretary of State.

Recommendation 73

The Council for the Regulation of Healthcare Professionals should have formal powers to require bodies which regulate the separate groups of healthcare professionals to conform to principles of good regulation. It should act as a source of guidance and of good practice. It should seek to ensure that in practice the bodies which regulate healthcare professionals behave in a consistent and broadly similar manner.

We agree. One of the functions proposed for the new Council is to ensure that the regulatory bodies act in a consistent manner, and it is proposed that it should have reserve powers so that it is able to fulfil its statutory functions. In exercising these powers the new Council will be expected to respect the independence of the regulatory bodies and allow them the maximum opportunity to act voluntarily.

Recommendation 75

Pilot schemes should be established to develop and evaluate the feasibility of making the first year's course of undergraduate education common to all those wishing to become healthcare professionals.

We agree. We are already piloting common learning undergraduate programmes. We will ensure that we develop and evaluate a range of workable approaches.

Recommendation 76

Universities should develop closer links between medical schools and schools of nursing education with a view to providing more joint education between medical and nursing students.

We agree. Universities are already developing closer links with schools of nursing education.

Recommendation 77

Universities should develop closer links between medical and nursing schools and centres for education and training in health service and public sector management, with a view to enabling all healthcare professionals to learn about management.

We agree. The NHS Leadership Centre will be working with medical and nursing schools to ensure management skills are developed within all programmes curricula for health care professionals.

Recommendation 78

Access to medical schools should be widened to include people from diverse academic and socio-economic backgrounds. Those with qualifications in other areas of healthcare and those with an educational background in subjects other than science, who have the ability and wish to do so, should have greater opportunities than is presently the case, to enter medical schools.

We agree. When medical schools were asked to bid for extra places in 2000 and 2001 they were asked to demonstrate an active commitment to recruiting students from a broad range of social, ethnic and educational backgrounds.

Recommendation 79

The attributes of a good doctor, as set down in the GMC's *'Good Medical Practice'*, must inform every aspect of the selection criteria and curricula of medical schools.

We agree. Planned improvements in selection criteria and medical schools' curricula will help to ensure that doctors develop the skills and attributes set out in the GMC's *Good Medical Practice.*

Recommendation 80

The NHS and the public should be involved in (a) establishing the criteria for selection and (b) the selection of those to be educated as doctors, nurses and as other healthcare professionals.

We agree in principle. All recruitment and admission procedures are based on published criteria to assist transparency, and ensure that selection is based on the applicant's ability and potential. We are committed to encourage broad participation in selection procedures.

Recommendation 81

In relation to doctors, we endorse the proposal to establish a Medical Education Standards Board (MESB), to co-ordinate postgraduate medical training. The MESB should be part of and answerable to the GMC which should have a wider role.

We do not accept the recommendation. Post-graduate training needs to take into account the needs of the service as well as the needs of individual clinicians. The MESB therefore needs to have closer links with the NHS.

Recommendation 82

CPD, being fundamental to the quality of care provided to patients, should be compulsory for all healthcare professionals.

We agree. It is already part of the duty of health care professionals to maintain their knowledge and skills and keep themselves up to date. This forms part of the appraisal and revalidation process.

Recommendation 83

Trusts and primary care trusts should provide incentives to encourage healthcare professionals to maintain and develop their skills. The contract (or, in the case of GPs, other relevant mechanism) between the trust and the healthcare professional should provide for the funding of CPD and should stipulate the time which the trust will make available for CPD.

We agree. £20 million is being invested this year to support implementation of appraisal and better access to CPD, with more to come in the next couple of years. We are clear, and this was emphasised in the NHS HR Performance Framework, that all health care professionals should have a personal development plan. In the case of doctors a formal PDP will be required as part of appraisal.

Recommendation 84

Trusts and primary care trusts must take overall responsibility through an agreed plan for their employees' use of the time allocated to CPD. They must seek to ensure that the resources deployed for CPD contribute towards meeting the needs of the trust and of its patients, as well as meeting the professional aspirations of individual healthcare professionals.

We agree. It has already been made clear that CPD requirements should be identified on the basis of the individual's needs, but in the context of the organisation's needs. The formal appraisal process should ensure that both professionals and their managers take appraisal and personal development seriously.

Recommendation 85

Periodic appraisal should be compulsory for all healthcare professionals. The requirement to participate in appraisal should be included in the contract of employment.

We agree. The Government has made clear that appraisal will be introduced for all health professionals. It is now being rolled out for all NHS doctors, having started with consultants on 1 April 2001. Work is underway to scope the implications of extending appraisal in a corporate way to all NHS staff. The scoping work was completed by the end of 2001 and we expect to make major progress in developing new systems by the end of 2002.

Recommendation 86

The commitment in *'The NHS Plan'* to introduce regular appraisal for hospital consultants must be implemented as soon as possible.

We agree. Consultant appraisal was introduced on 1 April 2001. GP appraisal is under negotiation. Appraisal for other doctors will be rolled out in 2002.

Recommendation 87

The requirement to undergo periodic appraisal should also be incorporated into GPs' terms of service.

We agree. GP appraisal is under negotiation following the same principles as consultant appraisal.

Recommendation 88

Periodic revalidation, whereby healthcare professionals demonstrate that they remain fit to practise in their chosen profession, should be compulsory for all healthcare professionals. The requirement to participate in periodic revalidation should be included in the contract of employment.

We agree. We are currently working with the GMC to introduce revalidation for all doctors. We will work with other regulatory and professional bodies to ensure a consistent approach for all health professionals.

Recommendation 89

The public, as well as the employer and the relevant professional group, must be involved in the processes of revalidation.

We agree. Medical revalidation will involve lay people participating in local panels. This will provide a benchmark for other professions.

Recommendation 90

The new Council for the Regulation of Healthcare Professionals should take as a further priority an early review of the various systems of revalidation and re-registration to ensure that they are sufficiently rigorous, and in alignment both with each other and with other initiatives to protect the public. The Council should also seek ways to incorporate managers (as healthcare professionals) into the systems of CPD, appraisal and revalidation.

We agree. The Council will have a critical role in ensuring consistency across the regulatory bodies. We will develop a code of conduct for senior managers.

155

The Department of Health's Response to the Report of the Public Inquiry into children's heart surgery at the Bristol Royal Infirmary 1984-1995

Recommendation 91

Managers as healthcare professionals should be subject to the same obligations as other healthcare professionals, including being subject to a regulatory body and professional code of practice.

We agree in part. We do not think it is practicable to establish self-regulation for senior managers. We do agree that the standards expected of senior NHS managers should be explicit. We favour a code of conduct, stronger performance management and tighter contracts rather than regulation.

Recommendation 92

Where clinicians hold managerial roles which extend beyond their immediate clinical practice, sufficient protected time in the form of allocated sessions must be made available for them to carry out that managerial role.

We agree. Under the Government's proposals for the new consultant contract, consultants' job plans will specifically address the time commitments needed for managerial duties.

Recommendation 93

Any clinician, before appointment to a managerial role, must demonstrate the managerial competence to undertake what is required in that role: training and support should be made available by trusts and primary care trusts.

We agree. Clinical director and medical director development programmes are to be rolled out from January 2002.

Recommendation 94

Clinicians should not be required or expected to hold managerial roles on bases other than competence for the job. For example, seniority or being next in turn are not appropriate criteria for the appointment of clinicians to managerial roles.

We agree. The values and behaviours framework for leadership is in the final stages of development and will be distributed to all Trusts by the end of February 2002. This will be applied to clinicians moving into managerial roles.

Recommendation 95

The professional and financial incentives for senior clinicians to undertake full-time senior managerial roles should be reviewed: the aim should be to enable senior clinicians to move into a full-time managerial role, and subsequently, if they so wish, to move back into clinical practice after appropriate retraining and revalidation.

We agree. Revalidation and recertification together with appraisal and better systems for professional development will make it easier to move between clinical and managerial roles.

Recommendations 96 and 97

To protect patients, in the case of clinicians who take on managerial roles but wish to continue to practise as clinicians, experts together with managers from the NHS should issue advice as to the minimum level of regular clinical practice necessary to enable a clinician to provide care of a good quality. Clinicians not maintaining this level of practice should not be entitled to offer clinical care. This rule should also apply to all other clinicians who, for whatever reason, are not in full-time practice, and not only to those in part-time managerial roles.

To facilitate the movement of clinicians in and out of managerial positions, the proposed systems for the revalidation (and re-registration) of doctors, nurses and professions allied to medicine should distinguish between professionals who are managers and also maintaining a clinical practice and those who are not. Those who are not maintaining a clinical practice should be entitled to obtain the appropriate revalidation (and re-registration to restart a clinical practice), after retraining, and should be assisted in doing so.

We reject. We do not believe it is possible to prescribe a minimum level of regular clinical practice to suit all specialties. When revalidating or re-registering, health professionals will need to provide evidence that they are competent to practise. Advisory and support services will be available as part of the appraisal process for those outside substantive employment.

Recommendation 98

The relevant professional regulatory bodies should make rules varying the professional duties of those professionals, whose registration they hold, who are in full-time managerial roles, so as to take account of the fact that, while occupying such roles, they do not undertake responsibility for the care of patients.

We reject. Most health professionals, even those in full-time management roles, need to retain their professional status. We do not believe it would be helpful to patients if registration status was subject to periodic changes.

157

The Department of Health's Response to the Report of the Public Inquiry into children's heart surgery at the Bristol Royal Infirmary 1984-1995

Recommendation 99

Any clinician carrying out any clinical procedure for the first time must be directly supervised by colleagues who have the necessary skill, competence and experience until such time as the relevant degree of expertise has been acquired.

We agree. Job plans for consultants include responsibility for the supervision of their staff as well as for themselves when carrying out procedures for the first time. The appraisal process for consultants, in place from April 2001, identifies professional development needs.

Recommendations 100 - 102

Before any *new* and hitherto untried invasive clinical procedure can be undertaken for the first time, the clinician involved should have to satisfy the relevant local research ethics committee that the procedure is justified and it is in the patient's interests to proceed. Each trust should have in place a system for ensuring that this process is complied with.

Local research ethics committees should be re-formed as necessary so that they are capable of considering applications to undertake new and hitherto untried invasive clinical procedures.

Patients are always entitled to know the extent to which a procedure which they are about to undergo is innovative or experimental. They are also entitled to be informed about the experience of the clinician who is to carry out the procedure.

We agree in principle. New interventional procedures will be overseen and scrutinised by NICE from April 2002. LRECs will need to consider any studies of new procedures as advised by NICE. Guidance on the new arrangements will specify local systems for managing new interventional procedures and will be issued in 2002. This guidance will make clear the information clinicians must give to patients about new procedures, including their own experience and how further information can be assessed.

Recommendation 103

The Royal College of Surgeons of England should, in partnership with university medical schools and the NHS, be enabled to develop its unit for the training of surgeons, particularly in new techniques. It should also explore the question of whether there is an age beyond which surgeons, specifically in areas such as paediatric cardiac surgery, should not attempt new procedures or even should not continue in a particular field of surgery.

We agree. We will review the need for further development of the RCS training unit, in the light of NICE guidance on training requirements for the new interventional procedures which they evaluate. We have asked the Paediatric and Congenital Cardiac Services Review Group to consider age limits for surgeons undertaking paediatric cardiac surgery, as part of its report to be published in 2002. We will then consider this for other specialties and new procedures.

Recommendation 104

In the exercise of their disciplinary function the professional regulatory bodies must adopt a more flexible approach towards what constitutes misconduct. They must deal with cases, as far as possible, at a local level and must have available a range of actions which both serve the interests of the public and the needs of the professional.

We agree. Disciplinary matters are best dealt with at local level. Guidance on dealing with disciplinary matters at a local level will be available. The NCAA has been set up to provide support and advice to Trusts and health authorities in dealing with doctors whose performance gives rise to concern. Where local action has been unable to resolve the problem the NCAA will be able to make an assessment of the doctor and to recommend an appropriate course of action. The aim is to secure the necessary improvement through training and development.

Recommendation 105

The need to involve the public in the various professional regulatory bodies applies as much to discipline as to all the other activities of these bodies.

We agree. The public needs to be involved in all aspects of the work of regulatory bodies. The Government's proposals for the new Nursing and Midwifery and Health Professions Councils include strong input to both policy and casework. Proposals for GMC reform envisage greater public involvement.

Recommendation 106

We support and endorse the broad framework of recommendations advocated in the report ' *An Organisation with a Memory*' by the Chief Medical Officer's expert group on learning from adverse events in the NHS. The National Patient Safety Agency proposed as a consequence of that report should, like all other bodies which contribute to the regulation of the safety and quality of healthcare, be independent of the NHS and the DoH.

159

The Department of Health's Response to the Report of the Public Inquiry into children's heart surgery at the Bristol Royal Infirmary 1984-1995

We reject the recommendation that the NPSA should be outwith the NHS. It was established in July 2001 as a Special Health Authority. This provides the independence necessary to give the Agency credibility with patients and the public while ensuring it has the confidence of health care staff and is able to work closely with the NHS.

Recommendation 107
Every effort should be made to create in the NHS an open and non-punitive environment in which it is safe to report and admit sentinel events.

We agree. The work of the NPSA together with the clinical governance initiative and the Department's Risk Management System aims to develop a 'just culture' where non-punitive reporting of adverse incidents will help to improve patient safety.

Recommendation 108
Major studies should, as a matter of priority, be carried out to investigate the extent and type of sentinel events in the NHS to establish a baseline against which improvements can be made and measured.

We agree. The system for establishing a national database of adverse incidents and near misses currently being piloted by the NPSA will provide the baseline against which future improvements can be judged. The pilots will be completed early in 2002.

Recommendation 109
There should a single, unified, accessible system for reporting and analysing sentinel events, with clear protocols indicating the categories of information which must be reported to a national database.

We agree. The new national reporting system will be rolled out early in 2002.

Recommendation 110
The national database of sentinel events should be managed by the National Patient Safety Agency, so as to ensure that a high degree of confidence is placed in the system by the public.

We agree. The new system will be managed by the NPSA. Patients and carers will be able to report events directly to the NPSA.

Recommendation 111

The National Patient Safety Agency, in the exercise of its function of surveillance of sentinel events, should be required to inform all trusts of the need for immediate action, in the light of occurrences reported to it. The Agency should also be required to publish regular reports on patterns of sentinel events and proposed remedial actions.

We agree. Guidance will make clear the appropriate local action needed in respect of any adverse incident which is reported to the NPSA. The NPSA will publish regular reports on trends and patterns and disseminate guidance on the lessons learned. Guidance is currently being piloted.

Recommendation 112

***All* sentinel events should be subject to a form of structured analysis in the trust where they occur, which takes into account not only the conduct of individuals, but also the wider contributing factors within the organisation which may have given rise to the event.**

We agree. This is already a requirement of the Department's Risk Management System. It will be reinforced by root cause analysis of serious incidents to understand the underlying cause(s). Guidance will be issued by the NPSA in 2002.

Recommendation 113

The reporting of sentinel events must be made as easy as possible, using all available means of communication (including a confidential telephone reporting line).

We agree. The aim is that most reports of adverse incidents to the NPSA will be transmitted electronically. A free-phone confidential telephone line will also be established.

Recommendations 114, 115 and 117

Members of staff in the NHS should receive immunity from disciplinary action by the employer or by a professional body if they report a sentinel event to the trust or to the national database within 48 hours, except where they themselves have committed a criminal offence.

Members of staff in the NHS who cover up or do not report a sentinel event may be subject to disciplinary action by their employer or by their professional body.

There should be a stipulation in every healthcare professional's contract that sentinel events must be reported, that reporting can be confidential, and that reporting within a specified time period will not attract disciplinary action.

We agree in principle, unless for example a criminal offence has been committed, and will be exploring, through the work of the CMO's Committee on Clinical Negligence, how this can be introduced.

Recommendation 116

The opportunity should exist to report a sentinel event in confidence.

We agree. Information reported to the NPSA will be held in confidence.

Recommendation 118

The process of reporting of sentinel events should be integrated into every trust's internal communications, induction training and other staff training. Staff must know what is expected of them, to whom to report and what systems are in place to enable them to report.

We agree. This will be included in the revised guidance on the Department's Risk Management System, to be issued in January 2002 and guidance from the NPSA.

Recommendation 119

In order to remove the disincentive to open reporting and the discussion of sentinel events represented by the clinical negligence system, this system should be abolished. It should be replaced by an alternative system for compensating those patients who suffer harm arising out of treatment from the NHS. An expert group should be established to advise on the appropriate method of compensation to be adopted.

We agree that the current system of clinical negligence compensation needs to be reformed. A White Paper will be published early in 2002 setting out proposals for reforms to the system. This will be informed by a committee, chaired by the Chief Medical Officer, which is reviewing all the potential options for reform.

Recommendation 120

The proposed National Patient Safety Agency should, as a matter of urgency, bring together managers in the NHS, representatives of the pharmaceutical companies and manufacturers of medical equipment, members of the healthcare professions and the public, to seek to apply approaches based on engineering and design so as to reduce (and eliminate to the extent possible) the incidence of sentinel events.

We agree. We are working with the Design Council to look at ways of improving safety of health care through new engineering and design solutions.

Recommendation 121

At the level of individual trusts, an executive member of the board should have the responsibility for putting into operation the trust's strategy and policy on safety in clinical care. Further, a non-executive director should be given specific responsibility for providing leadership to the strategy and policy aimed at securing safety in clinical care.

We agree in part. We believe that safety is an issue of such importance that it should be the responsibility of the whole board. We will however issue guidance requiring each Trust board to designate a non-executive director to provide leadership.

Recommendations 122 and 123

One body should be responsible for co-ordinating *all* action relating to the setting, issuing and keeping under review of national clinical standards: this should be NICE, suitably structured so as to give it the necessary independence and authority.

Once the recommended system is in place, only NICE should be permitted to issue national clinical standards to the NHS. The DoH (as the headquarters of the NHS) while issuing, for example, National Service Frameworks and supplementary guidance, should not be able to rescind or detract from the standards issued by NICE.

We reject. NICE is the foremost body in providing authoritative clinical guidelines and technology appraisals. However other bodies – MCA, MDA, NPSA, and the CMOs of the UK are still best placed to set standards in their fields.

Recommendation 124

NICE should pursue vigorously its current policy of involving as wide a community as possible, including the public, patients and carers, in the work to develop and keep under review clinical standards. In particular, the special expertise of the Royal Colleges and specialist professional associations should be harnessed and supported. Account should also be taken of the expertise of the senior management of the NHS.

We agree. NICE actively involves a range of stakeholders via six national Collaborating Centres and a special unit to help patients and carers who wish to participate in developing guidelines. NICE also seeks comments from NHS bodies on its draft recommendations.

163

The Department of Health's Response to the Report of the Public Inquiry into children's heart surgery at the Bristol Royal Infirmary 1984-1995

Recommendation 125

National standards of clinical care should reflect the commitment to patient-centred care and thus in future be formulated from the perspective of the patient. The standards should address the quality of care that a patient with a given illness or condition is entitled to expect to receive from the NHS. The standards should take account of the best available evidence. The standards should include guidance on how promptly patients should get access to care. They should address the roles and responsibilities of the various healthcare professionals who will care for the patient. They should take account of the patient's journey from primary care, into the hospital system (if necessary), and back to primary and community care, and of the necessary facilities and equipment.

We agree. NICE guidelines are developed to ensure that clinical standards are focused on the patient. Special versions of guidance are written for patients and carers.

Recommendation 126

Such standards for clinical care as are established should distinguish clearly between those which are obligatory and must be observed, and those to which the NHS should aspire over time.

We reject. Where NICE guidance exists it will become the standard. Advice from professional bodies which goes beyond NICE guidance may be regarded as aspirational.

Recommendation 127

A timetable over the short, medium and long term should be published, and revised periodically, for the development of national clinical standards, so that the public may be consulted and kept aware of those areas of healthcare which are covered by such standards and those which will be covered in the future. Target dates should be set by which clinical standards will have been prepared for all major conditions and illnesses.

We agree in principle. NICE already publishes a timetable for the production of its standards on its website. Furthermore we are publishing a consultation document covering the detail of the process of topic selection for NICE.

Recommendation 128

Resources, and any necessary statutory authority, must be made available to NICE to allow it to perform its role of developing, issuing and keeping under review national clinical standards.

We agree. Funding for NICE has grown in line with its increasing activity.
Legal changes to strengthen NICE's independence will be effected this year.

Recommendation 129

**Standards of clinical care which patients are entitled to expect to receive in
the NHS should be made public.**

We agree. NICE already publishes its guidance and produces versions tailored
to patients' and carers' needs.

Recommendation 130

**There must be a single, coherent, co-ordinated set of generic standards:
that is, standards relating to the patient's experience and the systems for
ensuring that care is safe and of good quality (for example corporate
management, clinical governance, risk management, clinical audit, the
management and support of staff, and the management of resources).
Trusts must comply with these standards.**

We agree. Clinical governance already provides a comprehensive framework
against which Trusts' services can be judged. In addition all Trusts are required
by the Treasury to maintain effective systems of financial, organisational and
clinical controls.

Recommendation 131-141

**The current system of inspection of trusts and primary care trusts should
be changed to become a system of validation and periodic revalidation of
these trusts. The system should be supportive and flexible. Its aim should
be to promote continued improvement in the quality of care.**

**One body should be responsible for validating and re-validating NHS
trusts and primary care trusts. This body should be CHI, suitably
structured so as to give it the necessary independence and authority.
Other bodies (for example the NHS Litigation Authority) which are
currently concerned with setting and requiring compliance with those
generic standards which should fall within the authority of CHI, should
carry out their role in this respect under the authority of and answerable
to CHI.**

**Validation and revalidation of trusts should be based upon compliance
with the generic standards which relate to the patient's experience and the
systems for ensuring that care is safe and of good quality.**

**The standards against which trusts are to be validated, and the results of
the process of validation or revalidation, should be made public.**

Any organisation in the voluntary or private sector which provides services to NHS patients should be required to meet the standards for systems, facilities and staff which organisations in the NHS must meet. The aim should be that, wherever care is funded by the NHS, there is a single system of validation which indicates to the public that the organisation meets the necessary standards.

The validating body should have the power to withdraw, withhold or suspend a trust's validation if standards fall such as to threaten the quality of care or the safety of patients. Any trust or organisation whose validation may be affected in this way must be given the opportunity to take appropriate remedial action. It must then satisfy CHI that it has taken remedial action before its continued validation can be confirmed.

CHI should consider how it might work with the providers of those programmes of accreditation already adopted by a significant number of trusts. In the future, where required standards are met, CHI should accept as part of its validation process the accreditation obtained through these programmes.

The process of validation of trusts should, in time, be extended to cover discrete, identifiable services within trusts. This extension of validation should first be piloted and evaluated.

The pilot exercise for this form of validation should include children's acute hospital services and paediatric cardiac surgery.

Should the pilot exercise be successful, the category of discrete services which should be a priority for this form of validation are those specialist services which are currently funded or meet the criteria for funding by the National Specialist Commissioning Group (the successor to the Supra Regional Services Advisory Group).

For discrete services, whether specialist services or otherwise, to be validated trusts they must be able to demonstrate that all relevant aspects of the service can *currently* be met, rather than that the trust *aims* to develop so as to be able to do so at some point in the future. Trusts which do not meet the necessary standards to ensure the safety of patients and a good quality of care should not be permitted to offer, or continue to offer, the relevant service.

We reject. We have carefully considered these recommendations about validation and revalidation but believe they could have a detrimental effect on the delivery of health services. We recognise that swift action is needed to tackle major problems and therefore propose to give CHI the power and responsibility to recommend special measures for Trusts which fail to meet standards. CHI will remain a non departmental public body but through the NHS Reform and Health Care Professions Bill we propose that its independence will be reinforced, by requiring it to make an annual report on the quality of services to NHS patients, which the Secretary of State will lay before Parliament.

Recommendation 142

Where the interests of securing quality of care and the safety of patients require that there be only a small number of centres offering a specialist service, the requirements of quality and safety should prevail over considerations of ease of access. It is and should be the responsibility of the NHS to assist patients, and their families or carers, with the cost of transport and accommodation when they have to travel away from home to receive specialist services. Such support should not be the subject of a means test.

We reject the proposal to extend the current Hospital Travel Cost Scheme, but we will encourage Trusts to use their discretionary powers to support families visiting relatives, including children.

Recommendation 143

The process of clinical audit, which is now widely practised within trusts, should be at the core of a system of local monitoring of performance. Clinical audit should be multidisciplinary.

We agree. Multi-disciplinary clinical audit is already a key feature of clinical governance.

Recommendation 144

Clinical audit must be fully supported by trusts. They should ensure that healthcare professionals have access to the necessary time, facilities, advice and expertise in order to conduct audit effectively. All trusts should have a central clinical audit office which co-ordinates audit activity, provides advice and support for the audit process, and brings together the results of audit for the trust as a whole.

We agree in principle. Each Trust has a lead individual with responsibility for clinical audit and all doctors are required to participate in clinical audit programmes. It is for individual Trusts to decide how clinical audit activity should be supported locally, as part of clinical governance.

Recommendation 145

Clinical audit should be compulsory for all healthcare professionals providing clinical care and the requirement to participate in it should be included as part of the contract of employment.

We agree. This is already being addressed for doctors through the introduction of appraisal as a contractual requirement and the impending introduction of GMC revalidation. Trusts are responsible for providing the time and resources to enable multi-disciplinary audit to take place.

Recommendation 146

The monitoring of clinical performance at a national level should be brought together and co-ordinated in one body: an independent Office for Information on Healthcare Performance. This Office should be part of CHI.

We agree. Proposals for an independent new Office for Information on Health Care Performance within CHI are included in the NHS and Health Care Professions Bill. Though the detailed remit and functions of the Office have yet to be finalised, the Office will collect, analyse, and publish reports on clinical and other NHS data. The Office will also develop a clinical audit programme (to include audits currently within the NICE work programme).

Recommendation 147

The Office for Information on Healthcare Performance should supplant the current fragmentation of approach through a programme of activities involving the co-ordination of the various national audits. In addition to its other responsibilities, the new system should provide a mechanism for surveillance whereby patterns of performance in the NHS which may warrant further scrutiny can be identified as early as possible.

We agree. The Office for Information on Health Care Performance should undertake this task. The assessment, commissioning and surveillance of clinical audit systems will be key functions of the Office.

Recommendation 148

The current 'dual' system of collecting data in the NHS in separate administrative and multiple clinical systems is wasteful and anachronistic. A single approach to collecting data should be adopted, which clinicians can trust and use and from which information about both clinical and administrative performance can be derived.

We agree. Those responsible for the separate administrative and clinical audit databases are already working together to develop an approach which will avoid duplication. Implementation of *Information for Health* will provide the basis for a single approach to collecting data for both clinical and administrative needs through the electronic patient record, which will be introduced by 2005.

Recommendations 149 and 150

Steps should be taken nationally and locally to build the confidence of clinicians in the data recorded in the Patient Administration Systems in trusts (which is subsequently aggregated nationally to form the Hospital Episode Statistics). Such steps should include the establishment by trusts of closer working arrangements between clinicians and clinical coding staff.

The Hospital Episode Statistics database should be supported as a major national resource which can be used reliably, with care, to undertake the monitoring of a range of healthcare outcomes.

We agree. A number of steps have been taken to engage clinicians with the value of the data recorded in the Patient Administration System and Hospital Episode Statistics. These include a major consultation on performance indicators, discussions with the BMA about how HES data can be used to monitor clinical quality and research into how HES can be used on a routine basis to identify areas of possible clinical concern.

We recognise the importance of HES as the key database to underpin the whole of the clinical governance programme for the foreseeable future. Our investment includes work on a new contract and tendering the service for supplying HES data. This will deliver improvements in service and create the opportunity to extend the scope of HES to include outpatient and accident and emergency data, and data from the private sector. We are working to make the HES data more accessible to those in the service and to link it with ONS mortality data to provide a more effective measured clinical outcome.

Recommendation 151

Systems for clinical audit and for monitoring performance rely on accurate and complete data. Competent staff, trained in clinical coding, and supported in their work are required: the status, training and professional qualifications of clinical coding staff should be improved.

We agree. A re-evaluation of the training infrastructure for clinical coders will commence in 2002. The results of this evaluation will lead to a range of measures to improve the training and career structure of clinical coders. These measures will begin to come on stream in 2003.

Recommendation 152

The system of incentives and penalties to encourage trusts to provide complete and validated data of a high quality to the national database should be reviewed. Any new system must include reports of each trust's performance in terms of the quality and timeliness of the submission of data. The systems within a trust for producing data of a high quality, and its performance in returning such data in a timely manner to the national database, should be taken into account in the process of validating and revalidating the trust.

We agree. For the first time, we will include a data quality indicator in the annual NHS Performance Indicators. CHI has also been looking at the quality of data available to Trusts in its regular reviews of clinical governance. In addition, the NHS Information Authority has been commissioned to develop a data quality strategy to support the NHS modernisation agenda by September 2002. This strategy will cover roles and responsibilities at all levels, training needs, making data quality an integral part of all data sets and collection initiatives and the feedback of data as a key driver to data quality.

Recommendation 153

At national level, the indicators of performance should be comprehensible to the public as well as to healthcare professionals. They should be fewer and of high quality, rather than numerous but of questionable or variable quality.

We agree. We have recently undertaken a wide ranging consultation with the NHS and public on which performance indicators should be published. In September 2001 we published 6 high level indicators against which acute Trusts were 'star' rated.

Recommendation 154

The need to invest in world-class IT systems must be recognised so that the fundamental principles of data collection, validation and management can be observed: that data be collected only once; that the data be part and parcel of systems used to support healthcare professionals in their care of patients; and that trusts and the teams of healthcare professionals receive feedback when data on their services are aggregated.

We agree. We are investing in the *Information for Health* Strategy. Electronic patient records will be available by 2005.

Recommendation 155

Patients and the public must be able to obtain information as to the relative performance of the trust and the services and consultant units within the trust.

We agree. Performance indictors for each Trust will be published soon. Further development work is needed before information can be published on services and particular specialties. The Office for Information on Health Care Performance will publish independent information on NHS performance. We wrote with the support of the BMA, to NHS consultants in December 2001 telling them of our intentions to use available data to publish performance information at consultant team level. We will work with the medical profession to improve local data collection.

Recommendation 156

As part of their Annual Reports, trust boards should be required to report on the extent of their compliance with the national clinical standards. These reports should be made public and be made available to CHI.

We agree. Trusts are already required annually to produce clinical governance reports and to report progress in implementing NSFs and NICE guidelines. These reports are both public and available to CHI.

Recommendation 157

The involvement of the public in the NHS must be embedded in its structures: the perspectives of patients and of the public must be heard and taken into account wherever decisions affecting the provision of healthcare are made.

We agree. The NHS Reform and Health Care Professions Bill contains proposals for the establishment of local Patients' Forums and a national Commission for Patient and Public Involvement in Health (CPPIH).

Recommendation 158

Organisations which are not part of the NHS but have an impact on it, such as Royal Colleges, the GMC, the Nursing and Midwifery Council and the body responsible for regulating the professions allied to medicine, must involve the public in their decision-making processes, as they affect the provision of healthcare by the NHS.

We agree in principle. Royal Colleges and other professional bodies are moving towards greater public involvement.

Recommendation 159

The processes for involving patients and the public in organisations in the NHS must be transparent and open to scrutiny: the annual report of every organisation in the NHS should include a section setting out how the public has been involved, and the effect of that involvement.

We agree. The annual Patient Prospectus will demonstrate how the public has been involved and the effect of that involvement. Every acute Trust will publish a Patient Prospectus from 2003.

Recommendation 160

The public's involvement in the NHS should particularly be focused on the development and planning of healthcare services and on the operation and delivery of healthcare services, including the regulation of safety and quality, the competence of healthcare professionals, and the protection of vulnerable groups.

We agree. The Health and Social Care Act 2001 places a duty on NHS bodies to involve the public in the planning and operation of health care services.

Recommendation 161

Proposals to establish Patients' Forums and Patients' Councils must allow for the involvement of the wider public and not be limited only to patients or to patients' groups. They must be seen as an addition to the process of involving patients and the public in the activities of the NHS, rather than as a substitute for it.

We agree. We propose that Patients' Forums will ensure that the public are able to become involved in NHS decisions.

Recommendation 162

The mechanisms for the involvement of the public in the NHS should be routinely evaluated. These mechanisms should draw on the evidence of what works.

We agree. We propose that CPPIH will identify and disseminate standards for the establishment, operation and evaluation of patient and public involvement and will submit regular reports to the Secretary of State.

Recommendation 163

The process of public involvement must be properly supported, through for example, the provision of training and guidance.

We agree. We propose that CPPIH will support patient and public involvement by setting standards, providing training and monitoring services from the patient's perspective.

Recommendation 164

Financial resources must be made available to enable members of the public to become involved in NHS organisations: this should include provision for payments to cover, for example, the costs of childcare, or loss of earnings.

We agree. Expenses will be paid to those who volunteer for Patients' Forums, PALS and CPPIH.

Recommendation 165

The involvement of the public, particularly of patients, should not be limited to the representatives of patients' groups, or to those representing the interests of patients with a particular illness or condition: the NHS Modernisation Agency should advise the NHS on how to achieve the widest possible involvement of patients and the public in the NHS at local level.

We agree. A national citizen leadership programme has been initiated to support patient representative organisations and PALS.

Recommendation 166

Primary care trusts (and groups), given their capacity to influence the quality of care in hospitals, must involve patients and the public, for example through each PCG/T's Patient and Advocacy Liaison Service. They must make efforts systematically to gather views and feedback from patients. They must pay particular attention to involving their local community in decision-making about the commissioning of hospital services.

We agree. We propose that Patients' Forums should apply equally to primary health care and to secondary care.

Recommendation 167

A National Director for Children's Healthcare Services should be appointed to promote improvements in healthcare services provided for children.

We agree. Professor Al Aynsley-Green was appointed as National Clinical Director for Children in July 2001.

Recommendation 168

Consideration should be given to the creation of an office of Children's Commissioner in England, with the role of promoting the rights of children in all areas of public policy and seeking improvements to the ways in which the needs of children are met.

173

The Department of Health's Response to the Report of the Public Inquiry into children's heart surgery at the Bristol Royal Infirmary 1984-1995

Healthcare would be one of the areas covered by such a commissioner. Were such an office to be created, we would see it as being in addition to, rather than in place of, our other recommendations about the need to improve the quality of leadership in children's healthcare services.

We are following with interest the developments in both Wales – where a Commissioner has already been appointed – and in Northern Ireland where there is a consultation underway on this issue. We are committed to learning all the lessons from these initiatives. Under the Care Standards Act 2000 the role of an independent Children's Rights Director has been created.

Recommendation 169

The Cabinet Committee on Children and Young People's Services should specifically include in its remit matters to do with healthcare and health services for children and young people.

We reject. We do not propose to change the remit of the Committee because it can and does consider health matters where appropriate.

Recommendation 170

Each health authority and each primary care group or primary care trust should designate a senior member of staff who should have responsibility for commissioning children's healthcare services locally.

We agree. During 2002, as new structures are developed, each PCG and PCT will ensure that a senior member of staff has designated responsibility for commissioning children's services. Strategic health authorities will need to have monitoring arrangements to ensure that appropriate commissioning of services for children is in place.

Recommendation 171

All trusts which provide services for children as well as adults, should have a designated executive member of the board whose responsibility it is to ensure that the interests of children are protected and that they are cared for in a paediatric environment by paediatrically trained staff.

We agree in principle and will consider how best to take this forward as the existing NHS structures are replaced during the Shifting the Balance of Power programme. When it is published, the National Service Framework for children's services can underline and clarify what the arrangements should be.

Recommendation 172

The proposed National Service Framework (NSF) for children's healthcare services must be agreed and implemented as a matter of urgency.

We agree. A Children's NSF will be prepared and published.

Recommendation 173

The NSF should include a programme for the establishment of standards in all areas of children's acute hospital and healthcare services.

We agree. The children's hospital services module of the NSF has been fast-tracked and will be published in 2002.

Recommendation 174

The NSF should set obligatory standards which must be observed, as well as standards to which children's services should aspire over time.

We agree. There will be obligatory standards.

Recommendation 175

The NSF should include incentives for the improvement of children's healthcare services, with particular help being given to those trusts most in need.

We agree. Incentives for the improvement of care will be part of the 'earned autonomy' programme for the NHS. We will be considering options relating to children's services.

Recommendation 176

The NSF must include plans for the regular publication of information about the quality and performance of children's healthcare services at national level, at the level of individual trusts, and of individual consultant units.

We agree. This will be considered as part of the NSF.

Recommendation 177

There must be much greater integration of primary, community, acute and specialist healthcare for children. The NSF should include strategic guidance to health authorities and trusts so that services in the future are better integrated and organised around the needs of children and their families.

We agree. The NSF will address the question of greater integration of services between the different sectors.

Recommendations 178-180

Children's acute hospital services should ideally be located in a children's hospital, which should be physically as close as possible to an acute general hospital. This should be the preferred model for the future.

In the case of existing free-standing children's hospitals, particular attention must be given to ensuring that, through good management and organisation of care, children have access when needed to (a) facilities which may not routinely be found in a children's hospital and (b) specialists, the appointment of whom in a children's hospital could not be justified given the infrequent call on their services.

Consideration should be given to piloting the introduction of a system whereby children's hospitals take over the running of the children's acute and community services throughout a geographical area, building on the example of the Philadelphia Children's Hospital in the USA.

We will consider evidence on service configuration through the development of the NSF.

Recommendation 181

Specialist services for children should be organised so as to provide the best available staff and facilities, thus providing the best possible opportunity for good outcomes. Advice should be sought from experts on the appropriate number of patients to be treated to achieve good outcomes. In planning and organising specialist services, the requirements of quality and safety should prevail over considerations of ease of access.

We will consider evidence on optimal workload in relation to outcomes in the Paediatric and Cardiac Congenital Services Review and in the NSF process.

Recommendation 182

Where _specialist_ services for children are concentrated in a small number of trusts spread throughout England, these trusts should establish Family Support Funds to help families to meet the costs arising from travelling and staying away from home. The Funds should be administered flexibly and should not be limited to those on income support or with low incomes.

We reject. See response to Recommendation 142.

Recommendation 183

After completion of a pilot exercise, all trusts which provide acute hospital services for children should be subject to a process of validation to ensure that they have appropriate child- and family-centred policies, staff, and facilities to provide a good standard of care for children. Trusts which are not so validated should not, save in emergencies, provide acute hospital services for children.

We agree in principle, but reject the concept of validation (see responses to Recommendations 131-141). The arrangements for inspection and performance management, which apply across the NHS, include children's services.

Recommendation 184

Children should always (save in exceptional circumstances, such as emergencies) be cared for in a paediatric environment, and always by healthcare professionals who hold a recognised qualification in caring for children. This is especially so in relation to paediatric intensive care.

We agree. Children should normally be cared for in a paediatric environment. This will be addressed in the NSF.

Recommendation 185

The 1991 standards for the numbers of paediatrically qualified nurses required at any given time should serve as the minimum standard and should apply where children are treated (save in emergencies). The standards should be reviewed as a matter of urgency to take account of changing patterns in the provision of acute healthcare services.

We agree. The 1991 standards for the numbers of qualified paediatric nurses will be reviewed in the NSF.

Recommendation 186

All surgeons who operate on children, including those who also operate on adults, must undergo training in the care of children and obtain a recognised professional qualification in the care of children. As a matter of priority, the GMC, the body responsible for the revalidation of doctors, should agree with the Royal College of Surgeons of England the appropriate number and range of procedures which surgeons who operate on children must undertake in order to retain their validation. This will have consequences for the way in which general surgery for children is organised.

We agree. We will work with the professional organisations to ensure all surgeons who operate on children are appropriately trained and undertake an appropriate number of procedures.

Recommendation 187

Parents should ordinarily be recognised as experts in the care of their children, and when their children are in need of healthcare, parents should ordinarily be fully involved in that care.

We agree. Parents should normally be fully involved in the care of their children and this will be reflected in the NSF.

Recommendation 188

Parents of very young children have particular knowledge of their child. This knowledge must be valued and taken into account in the process of caring for the child, unless there is good reason to do otherwise.

We agree. Parental knowledge of their children should be taken into account in caring for the child.

Recommendation 189

Children's questions about their care must be answered truthfully and clearly.

We agree in principle. However, parents need to be involved in decisions about what individual children are told.

Recommendation 190

Healthcare professionals intending to care for children should be trained in the particular skills necessary to communicate with parents and with children.

We agree. Health care professionals will be trained in communication skills. This will be achieved through changes in basic training and through continuing professional development. (See the response to Recommendation 2).

Recommendation 191

Healthcare professionals should be honest and truthful with parents in discussing their child's condition, possible treatment and the possible outcome.

We agree. The consent initiative will support health care staff, patients and their families in reaching decisions based on a full and honest appraisal of the information and facts available. A model consent policy and model consent forms were published in November 2001.

Recommendations 192-197

National standards should be developed, as a matter of priority, for all aspects of the care and treatment of children with congenital heart disease (CHD). The standards should address diagnosis, surgical and other treatments, and continuing care. They should include standards for primary and social care, as well as for hospital care. The standards should also address the needs of those with CHD who grow into adulthood.

With regard to paediatric cardiac surgery, the standards should stipulate the minimum number of procedures which must be performed in a hospital over a given period of time in order to have the best opportunity of achieving good outcomes for children. PCS must not be undertaken in hospitals which do not meet the minimum number of procedures. Considerations of ease of access to a hospital should not be taken into account in determining whether PCS should be undertaken at that hospital.

With regard to those surgeons who undertake paediatric cardiac surgery, although not stipulating the number of operating sessions sufficient to maintain competence, it may be that four sessions a week should be the minimum number required. Agreement on this should be reached as a matter of urgency after appropriate consultation.

With regard to the very particular circumstances of open-heart surgery on very young children (including neo-nates and infants), we stipulate that the following standard should apply unless, within six months of the publication of this Report, this standard is varied by the DoH having taken the advice of relevant experts: there must, in any unit providing open-heart surgery on very young children, be two surgeons trained in paediatric surgery who must each undertake between 40 and 50 open-heart operations a year.

The national standards should stipulate that children with CHD who undergo any form of interventional procedure must be cared for in a paediatric environment. This means that all healthcare professionals who care for these children must be trained and qualified in paediatric care. It also means that children must be cared for in a setting with facilities and equipment designed for children. There must also be access on the same site as where any surgery is performed to a paediatric intensive care unit, supported by trained intensivists.

Surgical services for children with very rare congenital heart conditions, such as Truncus Arteriosus, or involving procedures undertaken very rarely, should only be performed in a maximum of two units, validated as such on the advice of experts. Such arrangements should be subject to periodic review.

179

The Department of Health's Response to the Report of the Public Inquiry into children's heart surgery at the Bristol Royal Infirmary 1984-1995

We will consider. The Paediatric and Congenital Cardiac Services Review Group has been established to advise on these recommendations. It will report in 2002 and is required to recommend standards for this service. The work of this group will inform development of standards in the NSF.

Recommendation 198

An investigation should be conducted as a matter of urgency to ensure that PCS is not currently being carried out where the low volume of patients or other factors make it unsafe to perform such surgery.

We agree. A thorough review of services is currently underway.

The Report of the Public Inquiry into children's heart surgery at the Bristol Royal Infirmary 1984-1995: *Learning from Bristol.* (Cm 5207).The Stationery Office. July 2001.

Department of Health. *The NHS Plan: A Plan for Investment – A Plan for Reform.*(Cm 4818). The Stationery Office. July 2000.

Department of Health. *An Organisation with a Memory:* Report of an expert group on learning from adverse events in the NHS chaired by the Chief Medical Officer. The Stationery Office. June 2000.

Department of Health. *Reference Guide to Consent for Examination or Treatment.* March 2001.

Department of Health. *Consent: what you have a right to expect:* A guide for patients. July 2001.

Department of Health. *Consent: what you have a right to expect:* A guide for parents. July 2001.

Department of Health. *Consent: what you have a right to expect:* A guide for children and young people. July 2001.

Department of Health. *Consent: what you have a right to expect:* A guide for relatives and carers. July 2001.

Department of Health. *Removal, Retention and Use of Human Organs and Tissue:* Consultation on Draft Code of Practice on Families and Post Mortems; Model Consent Forms and Information Leaflets; Draft Interim Statement on the Use of Human Organs and Tissue. January 2002.

General Medical Council. *Tomorrow's Doctors.* 1993.

Department of Health/Department for Education and Employment/Home Office. *The Removal, Retention and use of Human Organs and Tissue from Post-Mortem Examination:* Advice from the Chief Medical Officer. The Stationery Office. January 2001.

Department of Health. *Reforming the NHS Complaints Procedure:* a listening document. September 2001.

Department of Health. *Shifting the Balance of Power within the NHS: Securing Delivery.* July 2001.

Department of Health. *Paediatric Intensive Care: "A Framework for the Future"* - National Co-ordinating Group on Paediatric Intensive Care – Report to the Chief Executive of the NHS Executive. July 1997.

Department of Health. *The New NHS: Modern, Dependable.* (Cm 3807).The Stationery Office. December 1997.

Department of Health. *A First Class Service – Quality in the new NHS.* Consultation Document. July 1998.

Department of Health. *The NHS Cancer Plan – A Plan for Investment, A Plan for Reform.* September 2000.

Department of Health. *Building a safer NHS for patients: implementing an organisation with a memory.* Report of an expert group on learning from adverse events in the NHS chaired by the Chief Medical Officer. April 2001.

Department of Health/National Patient Safety Agency. *Doing Less Harm: Improving the safety and quality of care through reporting, analysing and learning from adverse incidents involving NHS patients –* Key requirements for health care providers. August 2001.

Department of Health. *Appointments to the most senior posts in the NHS* (Executive letter EL(97)84). December 1997.

Department of Health. *Modernising Regulation in the Health Professions:* Consultation Document. August 2001.

Department of Health. *Meeting the Challenge: A Strategy for the Allied Health Professions – arts therapists, chiropodists & podiatrists, dietitians, occupational therapists, orthoptists, paramedics, physiotherapists, prosthetists and orthotists, diagnostic radiographers, theraputic radiographers, speech and language therapists.* November 2000.

Department of Health. *Making a Difference in Primary Care: the challenge for nurses, midwives and health visitors:* Case Studies from NHS Regional Conferences. March 2001.

Department of Health. *Making the change: A Strategy for the Professions in Healthcare Science.* February 2001.

Department of Health. *Agenda for change: Modernising the NHS pay system.* February 1999.

General Medical Council. *Good Medical Practice.* May 2001.

Department of Health. *Supporting doctors, protecting patients:* A consultation paper on preventing, recognising and dealing with poor clinical performance of doctors in the NHS in England. November 1999.

Department of Health. *Information for Health.* September 1998.

Department of Health. *Building the Information Core - Implementing the NHS Plan.* January 2001.

Department of Health. *A Commitment to Quality, a Quest for Excellence:* A statement on behalf of the Government, the medical profession and the NHS. June 2001.

United Kingdom Central Council for Nursing, Midwifery and Health Visiting. *Strategy for Public Involvement.* October 2000.

Printed in the UK for The Stationery Office Limited

On behalf of the Controller of Her Majesty's Stationery Office

01/02. 81709

183

The Department of Health's Response to the Report of the Public Inquiry into children's heart surgery at the Bristol Royal Infirmary 1984-1995

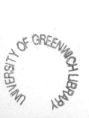